THE IRRITABLE BOWEL SYNDROME RELIEF

Seven Key Strategies to Conquer IBS

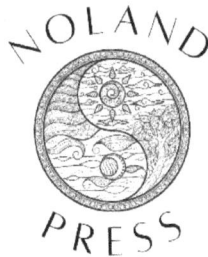

NOLAND PRESS

Joshua D. Noland

JoshNoland.com

IRRITABLE BOWEL SYNDROME RELIEF

Seven Key Strategies to Conquer IBS

Joshua D. Noland

ISBN: 978-1-965040-00-3

Stories and antidotes shared in this book are based on real people and situations. In some instances, names, places, and other details have been fictionalized to protect the anonymity of people discussed.

The information given in this book should not be treated as a substitute for professional medical or clinical advice; always consult a medical or clinical practitioner. Any use of information in this book is at the reader's discretion and risk. Neither the author nor the publisher can be held responsible for any loss, claim, or damage arising out of the use, or misuse, of the suggestions made, the failure to take medical or clinical advice, or for any material on third-party websites.

WHY THIS WORKBOOK

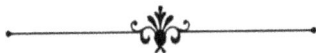

Are you seeking long-term solutions to conquer IBS? **Look no further.**

This book is your essential guide to understanding the science behind the root causes of IBS and offers proven methods to resolve your gut issues. By developing healthy habits and following the methods in this book, you can achieve lasting health and vitality. Discover the seven key strategies to overcome digestive distress and learn how to cultivate a lifestyle that supports your overall well-being. With these proven techniques, you'll gain control of your gut health and thrive.

ABOUT THE AUTHOR

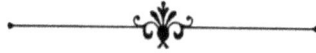

Written by Someone Who Has Personally Battled Irritable Bowel Syndrome and Discovered Lasting Solutions for Relief

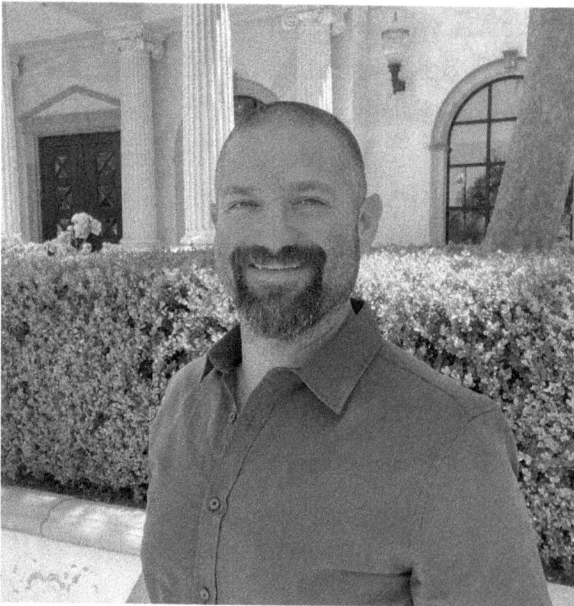

Joshua **D. Noland**, author, health coach, and chef, is passionate about helping individuals overcome their health struggles. He wrote this book to assist as many people as possible in finding relief from digestive distress. Through his research, Joshua has identified the correlation between the standard American diet and its impact on our bodies. His mission is to help people overcome their health challenges and live life to the fullest. Outside of his work, Joshua enjoys the outdoors, fitness, and adventure. Visit JoshNoland.com to learn more about him and access a wealth of free resources!

TABLE OF CONTENTS

FOREWORD

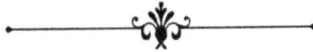

H ave you noticed that it seems like everyone is dealing with one or more health concerns? It seems that way because the majority of the population is indeed suffering from one ailment or another. Irritable bowel syndrome (IBS), Inflammatory Gut Disorder (IBD), celiac, leaky gut syndrome, and small intestinal bacterial overgrowth (SIBO) to name a few.

According to estimates from the National Institute of Diabetes and Digestive and Kidney Diseases, around 60 to 70 million Americans are affected by digestive diseases. That's approximately twenty percent of people in the U.S. which means one in five people are suffering with some kind of digestive condition.

These numbers are haunting and are getting worse every year. What is happening to our society? Have you seen those videos of school children in the 1950's, running, climbing across monkey bars, and doing jumping jacks? They are all in great shape, however the school children of today look much different.

One of the core issues concerning health today starts with the soil our food is grown in. It all comes down to the community of microorganisms that live in the soil known as the soil microbiome. These organisms consist of bacteria, fungi, protozoa, nematodes, archaea, algae, and micro arthropods. They break down organic matter into forms of nutrients plants can use and create pathways for water and air to get down through the soil to the roots of the plants.

When farmers till their fields, all of the microorganisms are killed and the nutrients of their carcasses will sustain plants with the nutrients they need for a while, but once they are all used up there is nothing left. This is when farmers use salt based chemical fertilizers. These fertilizers concentrate the salts in the soil over time and make the soil less and less productive.

At the same time farmers are practicing monocrop agriculture. This is the practice of growing only one type of crop in a field, it's efficient for harvesting but creates a buffet for pests. In turn, harmful pesticides must be sprayed to keep the pests at bay. These pesticides are poisons, and they can never be fully removed from the final product, and they affect your body negatively when we consume them.

If tilling wasn't bad enough for the soil micro biome, it also has to deal with weed killers like Roundup. This stuff is so toxic it kills all plant life including the vital microbes in the soil. They spray it on everything and not just once. Wheat is especially toxic because they spray it multiple times throughout the growing season and one more time right before the harvest to dry out the wheat.

Meat quality is also affected by poor land management and animal care practices. Ranchers let their cattle graze on grass until there is nothing left and then they move them to another pasture, degrading the quality of the soil. When they are old enough to provide enough meat to be profitable, they send them to a feed lot where the living conditions are horrible, and they're fed an unnatural diet of corn, soy, and waist products from other industries. This is all wrong and makes the cows sick.

Cows should be grazing on grass and moved often to help the quality of the pasture, It's called rotational grazing, and it sequesters carbon into the soil, improving the quality of the pasture and the end product. When cows are raised this way, they are healthier, and their meat is more nutrient dense. All animal operations should try to mimic the natural environment of the animals to produce the highest quality food and enrich the environment. They should also be treated with respect and if they do it right, they only have one bad day.

Monocrop agriculture damages the soil that provides the vital resources that plants need to grow nutrient dense foods and feed lot operations are producing sick and unhealthy animal foods, these practices are hurting the planet and us. We should be able to get all the vitamins and minerals we need from food but the food available in stores is not cutting it. We need to reshape our food system with regenerative practices, cover crops, crop rotation, and compost or other organic soil amendments.

Permaculture offers many regenerative techniques for growing plants and raising animals in ways that are harmonious with nature and provide the nutrient rich foods we need to thrive.

You can get higher quality foods and support local farmers and ranchers by sourcing your food locally. Talk to your local butcher and buy from farmers who practice regenerative and organic methods.

It's vital to support local food producers because having a decentralized food production system helps mitigate the impact of disasters on food production like floods or droughts. There are only ten companies that own almost all the big food brands around the world. These profit driven companies do not take health into consideration when making decisions on how to operate. This is a huge problem and when you support local food production you take dollars away from the mega corporations and give it back to your community, making it stronger providing you with high quality food.

Go to your local farmer's market, or visit your local rancher, to find the foods you need to heal your gut.

CHAPTER 1:
CLIMBING UP A LADDER:
HEARD SOMETHING
SPLATTER…

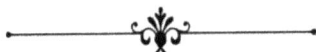

We had just finished brunch and were on the boat headed to the cove when the first cramp hit. I thought I would be okay since I had only eaten two pancakes, but then another stomach cramp hit me. *Oh no*, I thought. *This can't be happening, there's no bathroom on this boat!*

We were on vacation and had a whole day of adventure planned, however my stomach had other plans. I knew I had issues eating gluten, but I didn't care, we were on vacation after all. So, I ate whatever I wanted at brunch, and I paid for it once we got on that boat. I was so excited to go snorkeling and hang out on the beach but once that first cramp came, all my plans went overboard.

I asked the captain "How much longer until we get to the cove?" He said, "About 20 minutes." "Is there a bathroom," I asked. "No, but we do keep some toilet paper on board that you're welcome to use." At this point I knew what had to be done. I was going to have to shit in the jungle on some remote island and my fiancé would surely find out. Those twenty minutes felt like hours and as soon as we docked, I grabbed that toilet paper and dashed into the jungle.

"I hate that our trip ended early because I had so much diarrhea after brunch, but it made me realize that I have the power to change my situation by making better food choices." Barbara told her fiancé. "Damn those pancakes, damn them straight to hell."

Barbara and her fiancé's vacation was ruined due to her digestive issues, but on the flight home she realized that she had the power to heal her gut by eating the foods that served her body. One in five people are suffering just like Barbara and they have the power to heal themselves and you can too. More and more people are having digestive problems and doctors don't know how to help, like with many chronic illnesses today. Basically, it all comes down to lifestyle and the decisions you make that will have the most impact and I will help you get there.

Have you ever been in a similar situation to Barbara's? What would you be willing to do to solve this problem? Have you seen a doctor about your digestive problems, and if so, were they able to help you? I'm going out on a limb here and assume that they were unsuccessful and that's why you are reading this book.

In this book I will share with you the seven key strategies I used to heal my gut and find relief from irritable bowel syndrome. I'll get into the science of it all so you understand how it works and provide practical tips you can act on to reclaim your freedom from the porcelain throne. Developing a healthy lifestyle will significantly reduce the symptoms of IBS and allow you to enjoy life again. When you change your habits from ones that harm you to ones that serve you, it will make your daily routine your medicine. You don't need fancy treatments or expensive medicines. Mindset, diet, and activity can go a long way.

I didn't know I had IBS until I started learning more about it in recent years. I changed my lifestyle to lose weight and feel better emotionally, and as a side effect, my digestive issues vanished. A lot of people I know struggle with some kind of stomach issue and the ones who change their diet get better and the ones who don't just live with the pain and suffering. The seven strategies only work if you incorporate them into your daily routine and they become habit.

The seven key strategies to heal your gut are empowerment through education, personalized diet elimination, proactive nourishment, home-cooked healing, positive mindset, regular physical activity, and adequate hydration. There is no cure for IBS, but if you can master the seven key strategies you'll forget about IBS and can go on enjoying your life.

My whole life I've dealt with constipation, diarrhea, stomach pain and excessive flatulence. I never thought much about it. I would eat McDonalds and then my stomach would hurt for a bit. I would go to the bathroom, and I would feel better. I thought that's just how it goes. In high school, I would eat a personal pan pizza with a side of nacho cheese and a bag of

Flamin' Hot Cheetos for lunch almost every day, and I'd wash it down with a Coke. I didn't see anything wrong with that and I never realized how much it was affecting me until I started eating better.

In 2019 I got fed-up with being overweight and depressed, so I started talking to a therapist and started lifting weights a few days a week. I started to feel better, but I had a lot of weight to lose so I decided to start eating differently. I ate more meat and whole foods, and as a result, I ate less junk food. I replaced my evening candy binging with fruit and potato chips with homemade popcorn. Around this time is when my IBS symptoms started to disappear, and the weight really started flying off. It was hard at first but that feeling of not having to rush to the bathroom first thing in the morning and the additional energy I felt throughout the day was addictive. I was eating more whole foods and less processed foods, exercising, taking my mental health seriously, and loving life.

I was able to successfully incorporate the seven strategies into my daily routine and have been mostly symptom free for over five years now and I want to help you do the same. I have studied nutrition and how the body reacts to certain foods. I have a background in food service as a chef and I am personally familiar with the difficulties associated with emotional eating and food addiction. Changing what you eat can be very scary, many of us rely on food to comfort us and get us through a tough day, but once you find foods you enjoy eating and serve your body, you'll be golden. It takes time and it's not easy, but it is totally worth it.

This book offers proven and practical methods to win the battle taking place in your digestive tract. These methods have helped thousands of people and are backed by science. In the next chapter we'll discuss the technical aspects of bowel distress and the reasons why these methods work.

If you take this information to heart, I promise it will teach you how to take back control of your life. By following the methods laid out in this book you can heal your gut and overcome the debilitating effects of irritable bowel syndrome. I can give you the information, but only you can take the steps necessary to feel better.

We will do a deep dive into the seven key strategies to heal your gut and the 5R protocol in the upcoming chapters. First you will learn the science behind why this happens and why the strategies work. Then I'll go over the foods you should avoid during a major flare up and how to slowly start reincorporating foods to see which ones trigger you. We will review the foods you should include in your diet to avoid flare ups. I will also share a few easy recipes you can make to find relief during a major flare up. Did you know mindset plays a huge role in digestive distress? It does and I'll tell you how and some tips on turning that frown upside down.

By sharing the research that I have done on digestive issues and my experiences with them, I hope to spread awareness to those who are suffering and assume it's normal. I was able to resolve my symptoms and I know if you slowly start to implement the strategies in this book one at a time, you can be free from the IBS shackles too!

CHAPTER 2:
A SWING AND A MISS:
KNOWING IS ONLY HALF OF
THE EQUATION

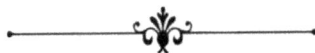

One second Bill was mid swing and the next thing he knew he was on the floor surrounded by people.

Bill was tired of getting the urge to go to the bathroom, only to discover that his bowels were not cooperating. He had been constipated for a few weeks now and nothing he tried had helped so he decided to go to the gym and get a workout in. He thought, *maybe if I get my body moving and my blood pumping, it might help get things moving.* He started his workout with a quick warm up and then moved on to kettle bell swings and that's when it happened. He was in the middle of his third swing, he started feeling dizzy, got disoriented, and ended up on the floor.

Bill was right, exercise can help with digestion but what he neglected to do was drink enough water. He knew that staying hydrated was a huge factor in constipation. His doctor had told him that a few days prior but there was a disconnect and Bill wasn't able to act on this knowledge.

Whether it's work, school, home, time with friends, or family, there is always something or someone that is seeking your attention and all of these things can distract you from taking care of yourself. Even if you know exactly what you need to do to fix your gut problems it's hard to forgo other activities to do the things necessary to heal yourself, but that is what it takes to get better.

You know when you're on an airplane and the crew does the pre-flight speech and tells you "in case of a loss in cabin pressure to put your oxygen mask on first"? This is how you heal your gut, by putting your health before your friends and family's needs. This can be easier for some more than others. Your family and friends will understand if you explain what you need to get better.

Mental health is the most important part of your healing process. If your head is not in the right place, you won't be motivated to make the necessary lifestyle changes and stick with them long enough to find relief.

Some people just deal with their health issues themselves until it gets so bad it's unavoidable, and they finally go see a doctor. Sadly, most doctors don't know how to treat the root causes of IBS and will either prescribe a drug or refer you to a gastrointestinal specialist (GI). They may request you get some blood work or give a stool sample, but most won't be able to give you a holistic solution to heal your gut. It's not their fault, it's just how they were trained to practice medicine.

The acronym "TOILET" can help us remember the

realities we will face when we're ready to truly heal the root causes of our digestive distress.

Time: It takes time.

Outings: The anxiety of planning outings around the proximity to restrooms and the challenge of avoiding foods that will trigger your symptoms.

Income: The impact on earning potential through missed workdays in addition to the added cost of medical care and treatments.

Lifestyle: The modifications needed in everyday life to manage symptoms.

Eating: Dietary restrictions and the constant need to be vigilant about what to eat.

Tension: The stress that comes with managing chronic symptoms can negatively impact your symptoms.

The solutions to resolve your IBS symptoms are simple but they are not easy. It will take time, knowledge, commitment, support, and a change in lifestyle. All these solutions if implemented will have numerous other positive impacts on your life besides repairing your digestive system.

Time:

Anything worth doing right takes time and healing your gut is no different. Your gut issues didn't happen overnight, it took years of eating ultra-processed foods, foods you're sensitive or allergic to, so it will take time to undo the damage. You may have noticed the symptoms appear overnight but most likely that was the tipping point.

Time is a tricky thing; we can't really grasp the true nature of time as it tends to change for us over our lifespan and even moment to moment. When you're not having fun because you're in pain from constipation, time seems to drag on and on. It is also interesting how when you start a new routine and get used to it, time can pass, and you forget that your new routine is actually new, and it becomes a part of your life. This is the goal with the strategies in this book.

You will have to be patient and working on your mental health will help you get there.

Outings:

The anxiety of planning outings around proximity to restrooms is a drag. Having to go to the bathroom so often can have a huge effect on what you do and where you go. Another aspect of outings is fitting in. Who wants to be that one person that keeps the group from going to that pizza place everyone is so excited to try because you can't eat pizza?

No one does, but it's part of the deal when you want to heal!

Finding foods that won't trigger your tummy to get upset while on an outing is challenging to say the least, but abstaining from participating in group activities may be required for a time.

Fitting in with a group is a survival skill but it won't serve you well if you have IBS, unless your group of friends all have IBS too and you can go places with ample bathrooms and lots of whole food options, prepared using clean cooking methods.

Income:

The impact on earning potential through missed workdays is a burden on your wallet and is sometimes unavoidable. You may have the additional expenses of medical care, medications, specialty foods, and treatments, and at the same time a loss of income due to missed days at work. Even if you have a job with benefits like health care and paid sick time nothing is free, and your sick time will eventually run out.

"Your lifestyle ultimately determines your health!"

Lifestyle:

You'll have to change your routine to manage your symptoms, a holistic approach is the only way to truly fix the root causes of IBS. Incorporating things like the low FODMAP diet, exercise, quality sleep, limiting alcohol, and meditation are some of the key practices you'll need to adopt to see real results.

Change is not easy, but it is the only constant in life. These changes will have positive health effects too like weight management and mood. As we grow older our bodies and minds change, and we need to adapt to these changes to stay relevant to the realities of our situations.

Eating:

Dietary restrictions, cravings, and social settings make eating the right foods for your stomach more challenging, and you will face many challenges during your path to recovery. Food is a huge part of culture and socialization. It sucks not being able to eat what everyone else is and it can make you feel isolated. If you take the time to explain your situation, your friends and family will understand, if not, maybe you need to reevaluate the people you surround yourself with.

Food is the only substance people are addicted to but cannot stop using. This presents a unique challenge. Most other substances people get addicted to are not required for survival, so you will need to approach this step carefully.

Tension:

The stress and mental or emotional strain that come with IBS can make your symptoms worse. It's a Catch-22, you're worried about what to eat and how it will affect your tummy but the more you do the more it negatively impacts your gut. This presents quite a challenge but it's manageable with meditation, mindset practices, and believe it or not, exercise.

If you don't act on the knowledge in this book, you may never know the peace of having regular bowel movements or be able to enjoy the foods that once triggered your gut distress.

> A long, long time ago in a far away place called Ohio, John was driving down a long stretch of highway in the middle of nowhere and all of a sudden, he felt the urge to go. His stomach cramped, he started sweating, and he had to go to the bathroom with a vengeance. There was nowhere to stop for miles, he had no choice but to hold it and fight through the pain until he got to a bathroom.

> John had been dealing with mixed IBS for five years. He had bouts of constipation for a while, and then he would have diarrhea for days on end. He never knew what

would trigger these alternating battles in his bowels.

He was over it; he had seen his primary doctor a few times and the GI specialist had recommended removing a huge part of his colon. John knew that surgery was only a last resort due to the risks involved and he knew it would not solve the root problem. The trouble was that John could not figure out what the root of his IBS-M was.

The surgery was scheduled, and John was reluctantly preparing for it. He arranged for a substitute teacher to cover his class and have someone care for his dog, Spike, and himself while he recovered for a minimum of six weeks. The surgery was only a week away and John really didn't want to go through with it, by chance he stumbled upon the "Meat Mafia" podcast and started listening to one of the episodes. The host was sharing their story of how they overcame ulcerative colitis by going on the carnivore diet.

John was desperate. *What do I have to lose?* He thought. So he went to the store, bought a bunch of ground beef and steaks, and started a meat-based diet. After a day or so he noticed his symptoms were not as severe and by the end of the week he actually started feeling better. John decided to cancel the surgery the day before it was scheduled, and he was thankful he made that decision because a year later his IBS-M symptoms were gone.

Have you ever experienced any hurtles when trying to identify the root cause of your IBS symptoms? Many people try to seek help either online or from healthcare professionals but if you are not committed to changing the way you approach your day-to-day life your chances for healing are slim to none.

"There is no pill that will fix you, recovery takes time and dedication."

If your doctor was unable to help you with your IBS, you are not alone. Approximately 40% of people who reported seeing their doctor for their IBS symptoms reported that traditional medical treatments did not adequately relieve their symptoms. According to the Cleveland Clinic, there is no way to prevent IBS, but I do not agree. We'll get into this in future chapters but for now just know many people are suffering with IBS and doctors who practice traditional medicine do not have much success treating it.

Doctors may be struggling to help their patients with IBS but there have been lots of people who were able to find relief. As long as you have an open mind and continue reading, you will discover what you need to do to heal. Once you finish this book you will have the knowledge you need, and it will be up to you to apply that knowledge to your everyday life.

You may be asking yourself, *Am I too old to benefit from these solutions? Has the window of opportunity passed me by?* If you are asking this question, the answer is a resounding "NO!" let me assure you, it is never too late to implement the solutions I present.

"How can I reduce stress when my IBS is stressing me out? Is it even possible? If this is a question you have been asking yourself the answer is Yes, it is possible! I and many others were able to overcome stress and anxiety and I will teach you how.

You may be wondering, *how am I going to pay for medical expenses when my symptoms keep me from going to work some days? How am I going to pay for expensive treatments and medications?* This is a huge concern for many suffering from IBS. Luckily, the solutions to treat your IBS symptoms are non-negotiable expenses like groceries and the rest of them are low to no cost.

What if my job requires me to go out late at night to socialize with clients? How am I supposed to get better sleep? How am I going to change my lifestyle? Some jobs may **"Your health must be your number one priority, if you want to truly get better."** present unique challenges and may be able to accommodate your situation if you ask. If not, then it may be in your best interest to start looking for another job.

It should now be clear that the power to change lies firmly in your hands. The strategies and insights shared in this book are more than just guidelines; they are the steppingstones to a new life, free from the shadow of irritable bowel syndrome. Imagine a day when you no longer plan around your symptoms, but instead, plan for your dreams. A life where discomfort and anxiety are replaced by comfort and confidence, allowing you to focus on the people and passions that truly matter to you. Let's embrace this new beginning with hope and step forward together into a brighter, healthier you.

CHAPTER 3:
SEVEN KEY STRATEGIES:
TO CONQUER IBS!

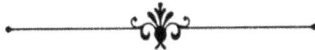

———————— ❦ ————————

There is no cure for IBS, however you can overcome its symptoms and sooth your gut with the tips and methods discussed in this book. Once your gut is healed you will be able to enjoy more foods and feel confident to participate in day-to-day activities without concern for where the nearest bathroom is. You will be able to enjoy eating again and have more energy.

The seven strategies to heal your gut have helped me and many others dealing with digestive distress and they can help you too. I promised that if you followed the advice in this book that you would find relief from your IBS symptoms, and these are the seven strategies that will get you that relief.

One: What is IBS

Understanding how Irritable Bowel Syndrome works and the root causes is the first step in finding relief from its symptoms and healing. You have to know why your body reacts the way it does to certain foods, so you can find ways to lessen reactions or stop them altogether.

There are many contributing factors that are compounded by

your life choices and the environment that lead to IBS and many other digestive syndromes. The word "syndrome" is more of a general term and refers to a group of symptoms that consistently occur together or a condition characterized by a set of symptoms, without necessarily implying a specific cause. In many cases, the exact cause of a syndrome might not be known, or there might be multiple contributing factors. Some syndromes have well-defined causes, such as genetic mutations or infections, while others may be the result of a combination of genetic, environmental, and lifestyle factors which is the case for IBS.

Two: Top Ten Foods To Avoid: During A Major Flare Up

When you are in the middle of a flare-up and everything you eat hurts your stomach you must avoid certain foods. The negative results of consuming these foods can vary from person to person, some more and some less, but it is recommended to abstain from eating them until you can get your gut to a place where it can function properly. Once your digestive system has calmed down you may be able to reintroduce some of these foods into your diet, but it all depends on how your body responds to them.

If you're in good health, your stomach may be able to deal with foods that aggravate it without causing you trouble, because your body has more resources to work with. So, the healthier you get the more options you will have.

Three: Top Ten Foods To Include: To Avoid A Major Flare Up

When you eat these foods, you will feel good and avoid major episodes. Foods with probiotics, enzymes, vitamins, and minerals help your body function properly. Fermented foods are a good example, and they are common among all traditional cultures because of the health benefits they offer when included regularly in your diet. Your gut microbiome plays a big role in your health and when you feed those little buggers what they need to thrive, so do you.

Bone broth is a game changer for digestive distress. It contains collagen and gelatin, which can help repair and support intestinal lining health. This is crucial for those who may have a compromised gut barrier.

Four: Recipes For Relief From A Major Flare Up

One of the most powerful things you can teach a person is how to cook. When you know how to prepare food you have the power to control all aspects of the process and you decide what ingredients to use and more importantly not to use.

I will teach you a few basic recipes that will give you relief during a major flare up and if eaten often can help avoid future attacks. These are simple recipes you can make at home using common home kitchen equipment.

Five: Stress and IBS: Get Your Mind Right

Have you ever heard of the vagus nerve? Are you familiar with the gut brain connection?

It's a very strong connection between your brain and your gut. There are over one hundred thousand neurons in your stomach and only ten thousand in your brain. The way you think can have an impact on your digestion, and the opposite is also true.

If you eat nourishing foods your brain works better. Scientists are still discovering exactly how this connection works in relation to other functions in the body, but the science is clear that there is a strong connection, and more research is warranted to discover all of the ways these connections work together in our bodies.

Six: Activity: The Missing Link

Living a sedentary lifestyle is the number one contributing factor to poor health after a poor diet. When you exercise your digestive system operates better and helps you to feel good emotionally. Everything you do has an effect good or bad, and when you are active it has a positive effect on your overall health.

When you feel good, you'll be motivated to maintain those feelings and you will be more likely to eat foods that help you rather than harm you. This positive cycle will keep you on an upward trajectory toward healing and getting back to doing the things that bring you joy.

Seven: Hydration

The human body is over seventy percent water and when you breathe, sweat, and digest food your body loses water to those processes. It's important to replace it with filtered water and electrolytes to keep your body functioning properly. If you are dehydrated, even in the slightest, it can significantly impact your digestive system and put unnecessary stress on your gut.

Your body needs water to produce saliva and stomach acid, both critical components of breaking down the foods you eat so your body can absorb the nutrients. This is one factor that most people do not consider, or if they do, they are missing the vital electrolyte component.

Drinking chlorinated tap water or beverages containing artificial ingredients may irritate your already inflamed gut and hurt your gut flora.

Chapter Summary

Are you excited about all the solutions that have been presented so far?

You should be!

It may take some time to incorporate them all and some effort, but these long-term solutions are what you need to get off the IBS bus and they will serve your overall health for the rest of your life.

So many of us suffer from constipation, diarrhea, bloating, gas, and upset stomach daily, but we don't have to suffer anymore. I have suffered from these ailments and occasionally still do, but as long as we follow the seven key strategies, we will feel better the majority of the time.

If you take this seriously these solutions will work for you unless you have other underlying health issues to address. The rest of this book is filled with the details on how to successfully execute the seven strategies. If you can successfully incorporate them into your lifestyle, you won't ever have to think about it again and that alone will go a long way in your recovery.

CHAPTER 4
WHAT IS IBS:
THE SCIENCE OF
GASTROINTESTINAL
DISORDERS

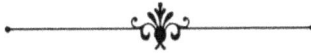

———————— ⚜ ————————

My social life is over, I'm going to have to become a recluse to avoid the embarrassment of always having major gas. She thought.

Emma, a young graphic designer, struggled with bloating and excessive flatulence. Her days were clouded in discomfort and anxiety, she never knew when the next flare up would strike. Emma felt powerless, as each meal felt like a gamble.

Determined to reclaim her life, Emma delved into research about gut health. She learned about the importance of eating a balanced diet, stress management, and regular exercise. Armed with this knowledge, Emma adjusted her diet to include more whole foods, fiber-rich foods, and some fermented foods.

She also embraced yoga and meditation, which not

only alleviated her stress but soothed her symptoms significantly. Gradually, her flare-ups became less frequent and less severe, and she felt a new sense of control and confidence.

Thanks to Emma's newfound knowledge she was able to make the lifestyle changes that gave her the relief that she desperately craved and the freedom to escape her cave of solitude. Her story is a testament to the power of education and personal determination in facing health challenges.

Have you ever felt like Emma did? It can be overwhelming and frustrating, especially if you don't know what the root causes are.

Knowledge is power is an underappreciated statement. With the internet at the tip of our fingers there is so much information it can be challenging to weed through it all to find the helpful information that is hiding amongst the nonsense.

I am going to share the knowledge I have gained about IBS with you throughout this book, however this chapter is going to focus on what IBS is and what causes it.

Some readers may be asking "What is the root cause of irritable bowel syndrome?"

There is not one root cause of IBS, it involves a combination of several factors, including abnormalities in gastrointestinal motility (the movement of the digestive system), visceral hypersensitivity (heightened sensitivity to pain in the gut), inflammation, changes in gut microbiota, genetics, and psychosocial factors such as stress and anxiety. These factors can vary from person to person, and the interplay between them likely contributes to the development and exacerbation of symptoms.

"UNWELL" is the perfect acronym to describe the root causes of IBS because when you don't take care of your body you become unwell and more susceptible to IBS.

Unmoving: Sedentary lifestyle.

Neglect Sleep: Not getting enough quality sleep.

Wrong diet: Eating foods that trigger your IBS.

Emotional: Stress from work, school, or other worries can worsen your symptoms

Limited knowledge: Not knowing how to heal or what your triggers are.

Low hydration: Poor hydration practices leading to slowed digestion and constipation.

Unmoving

This refers to your overall activity level and includes things like going for walks after meals or walking a minimum number of steps a day.

Neglect sleep

Sleep is critical for overall health and when your body is well rested, it has more resources to do what it needs to do. Getting quality sleep is important, too.

Wrong diet

Eating ultra processed food products or foods that are wrong for your body are the leading causes of IBS and most of the other digestive disorders. If you can identify the foods that trigger it and not eat them your gut will thank you and you will feel better.

Emotional

When you are stressed out about work, school, or finding the nearest bathroom, it causes havoc on your body. Having poor mental health or a negative mindset will only worsen your symptoms. In chapter eight I will give you practical methods to improve your outlook on life.

Limited knowledge

Being unfamiliar with what foods trigger or what foods soothe you can make or break you.

Low hydration

Your gut runs on water and when you are dehydrated it has a ripple effect throughout your entire body affecting all of its systems and functions negatively.

Other Digestive Disorders:

Inflammatory Bowel Disorder (IBD)

Ulcerative colitis

Celiac

Leaky gut syndrome

Small intestinal bacterial overgrowth (SIBO)

Crohn's

Diverticulitis

These conditions can be categorized as follows:

Functional:	Inflammatory:	Autoimmune:
❖ Irritable Bowel Syndrome ❖ Inflammatory Bowel Disorder	❖ Ulcerative Colitis ❖ Crohn's Disease ❖ Diverticulitis	❖ Celiac Disease ❖ Small intestinal bacterial overgrowth ❖ Leaky Gut Syndrome

Each category has different underlying mechanisms, but the solutions to find relief all remain the same with a few additional treatments when appropriate.

There are four different types of IBS based on symptom patterns.

The Four Main Subtypes of IBS:

IBS with constipation (IBS-C):

Characterized by predominantly constipation symptoms, such as infrequent bowel movements and difficulty passing stools.

IBS with diarrhea (IBS-D):

Characterized by predominantly diarrhea symptoms, such as frequent bowel movements and loose or watery stools.

Mixed IBS (IBS-M):

>Characterized by alternating periods of constipation and diarrhea, with no clear predominance of one over the other.

Unsub-typed IBS (IBS-U):

>Characterized by symptoms that do not fit clearly into the above categories or fluctuate between them.

These classifications can help guide treatment approaches, but it's important to note that individuals with IBS may experience symptoms from multiple subtypes or have symptoms that change over time. Luckily for you the solutions presented in this book will help no matter the subtype.

Traditional treatment methods are directed at treating the symptoms, not the root cause.

"If you see bodies floating down the river, you can keep pulling them out, but eventually, you need to go upstream to find out why they're falling in."

Meaning, we have to find the source of the issue. Doctors are trained to prescribe drugs to alleviate symptoms, not investigate the root cause. That's why the traditional medical approach does not work well for IBS.

What Is The Gut Microbiome?

What does my gut microbiome have to do with my gut issues?
You may be asking yourself this question and it's a good one.

The gut microbiome, also known as your intestinal flora, gut microbiota, or microbes, is a complex community of microorganisms, including bacteria, viruses, fungi, and other microbes, that live in the large intestines. This microbial community is highly diverse, hosting hundreds to thousands of different species that play critical roles in many aspects of health.

Functions of the Gut Microbiome

Digestion: Helps break down complex carbohydrates and fibers that our bodies cannot digest on their own. This process results in the production of short-chain fatty acids, which are important energy sources for the body and can influence metabolic health.

Immune System Modulation: The gut microbiome is essential in developing and maintaining the immune system. It helps teach the immune system to differentiate between harmful pathogens and harmless entities, thereby preventing an overactive immune response.

Protection Against Pathogens: By occupying space and using available nutrients, the beneficial microbes in the gut can help prevent colonization by harmful pathogens.

Synthesis of Vitamins: Some gut bacteria are capable of synthesizing vitamins, such as vitamin K and some B vitamins, which are important for various bodily functions including blood coagulation and energy production.

Influence on Mental Health: Research suggests a connection between the gut microbiome and the brain, often referred to as the "gut-brain axis." The microbiome can influence brain health and behavior, potentially affecting mental health conditions such as depression and anxiety.

A balanced gut microbiome is crucial for good health. When you eat processed foods, take certain medications, like antibiotics, or drink alcohol, you can cause harm to this community and your overall health. Eating a diverse diet rich in whole foods, reducing stress, and avoiding unnecessary antibiotics can help maintain a healthy gut microbiome.

Understanding the gut microbiome is a growing area of research, with implications for treating many diseases. For now, we know it plays a huge role in total body health and can be improved by eating fermented foods and whole foods. In extreme cases people do fecal transplants from a donor with a healthy gut microbiota to help repopulate an unhealthy one.

Your gut flora is closely linked to the microbiome of the soil. Remember in the foreword when I spoke about how current farming methods are hurting the soil microbiome? Well, this is affecting your gut flora and choosing to eat organic or home-grown foods, especially in their raw form will help strengthen your gut flora.

Gut Brain Axis

The stomach is known as the second brain because it contains neurons just like the brain does and it can have an influence on your emotions and more. This is where having a gut feeling about something comes from, your gut can literally communicate information to your brain. The gut actually has twice as many neurons as the brain and communicates information back and forth via the vagus nerve. This nerve runs from the brain to the heart, lungs, and the digestive system. It's a significant part of the autonomic nervous system, which controls involuntary bodily functions like heart rate, digestion, and respiratory rate. The vagus nerve is particularly known for its role in the parasympathetic nervous system, which is sometimes referred to as the "rest and digest" system. It helps to calm the body down after periods of stress.

The gut produces a substantial number of neurotransmitters, including about ninety percent of the body's serotonin, which influences mood and emotional well-being. It also produces other hormones involved in hunger signaling and digestion that can affect brain function.

When the vagus nerve transmits signals to the brain, especially the brainstem and areas involved in autonomic control and mood regulation, the brain processes these inputs and responds accordingly. This can affect feelings of hunger and satiety, mood, and even responses to stress. The brain can also send signals back to the gut via the vagus nerve to influence gastrointestinal function, completing a feedback loop that helps regulate digestion, immune response, and overall well-being.

This complex interaction not only helps manage basic bodily functions but also implies that our digestive system plays a crucial role in our emotional and mental health, highlighting the importance of maintaining a healthy gut and mind.

Age and IBS

The effects of IBS can change over time due to several factors. Changes in our behavior affect how our bodies respond to external stresses. The foods we eat, activity levels, and stress all play a part.

As we grow older our lifestyles continue to change, this can include changes in eating habits, living situations, and energy and stress levels.

The effects of the hormonal changes women go through during menopause can cause an increase in IBS symptoms. Luckily after menopause, symptoms tend to lessen in most women.

As we all get older our digestive systems may become more sensitive to certain foods as well. This is why you must take the advice in this book to heart and start implementing and incorporating the strategies into your life now, so you will be more resilient when things do change.

"Gut health should be your main focus to relieve your IBS symptoms."

How to break an irritable bowel syndrome cycle

The five R protocol is a holistic, multidimensional, functional medicine approach to gut repair. The five Rs are Remove, Replace, Re-inoculate, Repair, and Rebalance. By following this protocol, you can find relief from IBS and most of the other digestive disorders without taking dangerous medications like steroids and autoimmune suppressants or getting your colon removed.

Breakdown of the five Rs:

Remove: Stop eating foods that you are reactive, sensitive, intolerant, or allergic to. This can be accomplished by doing an elimination diet. Removing these foods will start the healing process and allow the microbes that feed on these foods to reduce in numbers which will also luckily lessen your cravings for them.

Replace: Replace those foods you were reactive, sensitive, intolerant, or allergic to with foods that nourish your body and help with healing. I have a whole chapter on this further in the book but bone broths or whole foods that are low in FODMAPs are a good place to start.

Re-inoculate: You know how important your gut health is and how your gut flora plays a critical role in this so you will need to get rid of the bad microbes and repopulate your gut with the good microbes by eating fermented foods and taking quality probiotic supplements.

Repair: Once you stop eating foods that irritate your gut you will need to let it recover by eating demulcent herbs (marshmallow root, slippery elm, and licorice root), probiotics, antioxidants, and foods rich in nutrients and enzymes. Fasting can help in this stage as well.

Rebalance: You will need to change your lifestyle to heal and stay healthy. Take advantage of all the health benefits that come with exercise, good sleep, and low stress. These things will not only fix your digestive distress but will give you a fuller and happier existence.

Chapter Summary:

Before I changed my eating habits and the way I cared for my body I was known in my household for my excessive flatulence, I had loose stools, and stomach aches daily. I thought it was just how it was, however after I stopped binging on junk food every night, eating fast food every day, and started focusing on my physical fitness and mental health, my symptoms went away. It was only after I got better that I realized I had suffered from IBS due to the foods I was eating and the lifestyle I was living.

Everyone's body reacts differently, some have minor symptoms, some develop major symptoms over time, and others can have a severe onset of symptoms overnight. No matter how you got here, I will give you the tools you need to heal and feel good again.

If you commit to following the strategies in this book including the five R protocol and take your health seriously you can conquer IBS and take back your life. The solutions are simple, but you must apply them to your everyday routine and make them habits to find lasting success and if you do you will get your health back and keep it!

CHAPTER 5:
TOP TEN FOODS TO AVOID:
During a Major Flare Up

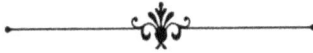

"My GI told me that what I ate had no effect on my IBS." This is unfortunately the kind of nonsense some doctors who are uneducated in bowel disorders will tell you but it's not true. Think about it, how can putting so much of a foreign substance in your body not have an effect, good or bad. The point is what you eat affects you and there are foods that will make it worse and foods that can help put the fire out.

I just can't do this it's too much! Barbara thought.

She had only been home a few days from her trip and was reading a book about IBS. She had come to the realization on the flight home that she could heal her gut, if only she could overcome her cravings for Flamin' Hot Cheetos, her favorite snack. Barbara was an emotional eater and when things got tough or stressful, she would eat to make herself feel better and her go-to snack was killing her. The book said she would have to give up processed foods and that included Flamin' Hot Cheetos, Barbara had a hard time dealing with this fact.

She had been to the doctor several times and her GI specialist told her "I want to put you on corticosteroids to bring the inflammation down."

Barbara responded "I'm worried about the negative side effects they could have on me like osteoporosis, high blood pressure, and mood swings."

"That is the price you may have to pay." Her doctor said.

That's crazy! Barbara thought and right then and there she made a commitment to herself to avoid the foods listed in the book for at least thirty days to see how she felt.

Food is one of the few things we can become addicted to that we can't quit; we all have to eat and most of us are emotional eaters like Barbara. I am and I struggle with the urge to splurge when I'm feeling down, tired, sad, or just bored.

Can you relate to Barbara? Do you struggle with emotional eating?

It's very common and it's easy to rationalize how a Twinkie might make you feel better in the moment after having a bad day, but in the long run that Twinkie will only hurt you and make you feel bad physically and emotionally. With a little effort, time, and practice you can overcome these urges and get on the road to wellness by avoiding the top ten foods listed in this chapter.

Elimination Diets

I was able to overcome most of my cravings for junk food and identify the foods I'm sensitive to by doing an elimination diet. I chose to try the carnivore diet (animal based foods only) and I did it in January 2024 for World Carnivore Month. I chose this particular elimination diet because it's simple, I was already eating a lot of protein, and I enjoy eating meat, so it was a no brainer for me.

What is an elimination diet?

Elimination diets are often used to help individuals identify food triggers. These diets involve removing specific foods or food groups from the diet for a period of time (fourteen to thirty days) and then systematically reintroducing them to see which cause symptoms.

Elimination diets are served best when you keep a journal of everything you eat, your bowel movements, and how you feel.

Having this data can help you pinpoint the specific triggers that effect your symptoms.

Pro Tip: Taking pictures of everything you eat can be an easy way to keep a food log. The pictures are date and time stamped so you can look back at the photos to correlate what you ate and how it affected you.

By doing an elimination diet for thirty days I was able to successfully kick some of the unhealthy food addictions I was dealing with and reduce my IBS symptoms.

The carnivore diet may not be right for you, fortunately there are several elimination diets you can choose from to help find relief.

Common Elimination Diets for IBS:

- ✓ Autoimmune Paleo
- ✓ Bone Broth
- ✓ Grain and Lactose Free
- ✓ LOW FODMAP
- ✓ No-Carbohydrate

LOW FODMAP

FODMAP stands for: Fermentable Oligosaccharides, Disaccharides, Monosaccharides and Polyols.

It's way more than just a diet, it's a classification of foods that are all short-chain carbohydrates (sugars) that are poorly absorbed in the small intestine. When these carbohydrates reach the large intestine, they ferment and produce gas causing bloating, constipation, and you guessed it, diarrhea. These foods are also osmotic, meaning they draw water into the bowel.

Oligosaccharides:

Are found in foods like beans and onions, they consist of a few monosaccharides linked together and are not as sweet as simple sugars.

Disaccharides:

A well-known disaccharide is sucrose, also known as ordinary table sugar, made from glucose and fructose. They are made when two monosaccharides are joined together.

Monosaccharides:

Fructose is one example of a monosaccharide and occurs naturally in fruits, some vegetables, honey, and other plants. Think of these as the simplest form of sugar and the basic building blocks for other types of sugars.

Polyols:

Examples of polyols include xylitol and sorbitol, often used in sugar-free food products. They are also known as sugar alcohols. These are sweeteners but they aren't as sweet as regular sugar and have fewer calories. Polyols don't spike your blood sugar like regular sugar because the body doesn't absorb them completely.

This diet is the most confusing of all diets but is the most scientific and beneficial for people who suffer with IBS. It's confusing because it's not clear cut, as some foods that are low in FODMAPs are okay in small quantities but if you eat too much, they can mess you up. You will have to memorize or refer to lists of foods that are okay for this particular elimination diet.

Even though this diet may be confusing at first once you get the hang of it, you could have much relief by avoiding high FODMAP foods.

Additional Low FODMAP Diet Resources:

Fodmapedia
(www.Fodmapedia.com/index-en)

This is a food database and indicates the level of FODMAPs in hundreds of foods. Free for everyone, but premium members have access to a larger number of ingredients and more detailed ingredient sheets.

The free service is good, but the premium has so much more information. It's relatively inexpensive at $4 a month or $40 a year.

You can try it out for free by going to: www.fodmapedia.com/free-trial-en

FODMAP Checker
(www.fodmapchecker.com/)

FODMAP checker is another food database, but it is very simple and will only show a check for foods low in FODMAPs or an X for foods high in FODMAPs. It is free and easy to use.

The good news is once your gut is better you may be able to enjoy whole foods that are higher in FODMAPs again.

Autoimmune Paleo

The Autoimmune Paleo (AIP) diet is an elimination and reintroduction protocol designed to reduce inflammation in the gut, heal the gastrointestinal tract, and subsequently decrease overall systemic inflammation. Although primarily targeted at autoimmune diseases, it is very effective for irritable bowel syndrome. The AIP diet is a specialized version of the original Paleo diet, which specifically aims to restore balance to the gut microbiota while optimizing overall nutrient intake.

The focus of the AIP diet is on removing foods that are commonly associated with sensitivities in order to lower overall inflammation.

The AIP diet includes:

- ✓ Coconut (oil, milk, flour, and aminos).
- ✓ Fermented food (kefir, kombucha, coconut yoghurt, kimchi, and sauerkraut).
- ✓ Fresh fruit (I would suggest removing fruits high in FODMAPs).
- ✓ Organic grass-fed meat, organ meat, and poultry.
- ✓ Seafood.
- ✓ Vegetables except nightshades.

Learn more about the autoimmune paleo diet at: https://mindd.org/diet/autoimmune-paleo-diet/

Bone Broth Diet

Homemade bone broth is the best thing for you when you have tried everything else, and your stomach is extremely sensitive. The collagen and gelatin in the broth sooth and heal your gut mucosal lining, the fat and protein fuel you, while the vitamin and minerals nourish your cells.

The best thing about making bone broth at home is you can customize it for your specific needs. You can use beef, chicken, pork, or fish, and you can make it as simple as bones, salt, and water. In chapter seven, I will provide a simple bone broth recipe.

Going on a bone broth diet for three to five days is a great way to sooth your gut enough so it can start healing and then go on one of the other elimination diets. This is my number one recommendation when you're in the middle of an attack and anything you eat makes it worse.

No-Carbohydrate Diet

This one is simple and straight forward but very limited in what you can eat. It comes down to meat, poultry, fish, and eggs. It most resembles the carnivore diet. If you can stick with a diet like this, you will reap the benefits of much more than just healing your digestive tract.

This is the elimination diet I recommend. After a few days of only drinking bone broth, I would move on to eating lean ground beef with only salt as the seasoning. If your system is okay with this, start adding lean cuts of beef like top sirloin or bottom round.

Grain and Lactose-Free Diet

The grain and lactose-free diet is similar to the no-carb diet, but it allows fruits and vegetables. This is a good option for most people as it still allows for a variety of different foods and is easy to classify what is or is not ok to eat. I would still recommend sticking with fruits and vegetables that are low in FODMAPs.

THE TOP TEN FOODS TO AVOID:

1. Ultra-Processed Food Products
2. Fats
3. Sweeteners
4. High Fructose Fruits
5. Certain Vegetables
6. Dairy Products
7. Legumes
8. Grains
9. Certain Beverages
10. Eggs

One: Ultra-Processed Food Products

If all you did was cut out all ultra-processed food products from your diet you would most likely cure most, if not all of the metabolic diseases you are suffering from including diabetes, high blood pressure, obesity, and yes, of course, IBS.

> ## Ultra-Processed Vs. Processed Food:
>
> Processed foods are altered from their natural state through methods like cooking or anything you do to prepare them to eat, and typically contain added ingredients such as salt or sugar but remain relatively close to their original form.
>
> Ultra-processed food products, however, undergo extensive industrial processing and include numerous additives like artificial flavors and preservatives, making them more convenient but less nutritious and even harmful to health. They do not even meet the definition of food and should be avoided at all costs if you care about your health.

According to The American Heritage Dictionary of the English Language, 5th Edition the definition of food is:

"Material, usually of plant or animal origin, that contains or consists of essential nutrients, such as carbohydrates, fats, proteins, vitamins, or minerals, and is ingested and assimilated by an organism to produce energy, stimulate growth, and maintain life."

According to this definition ultra-processed food products

do not qualify as foods because they are stripped of the vital nutrients we require to function. This is so they last longer on store shelves. Even worse these products are enriched with synthetic vitamins and minerals that our bodies can't use and may even cause harm.

The "natural" and artificial flavors in these foods mess with your body's natural ability to crave the nutrients it needs and leave it depleted and confused. Not to mention the artificial sweeteners and added sugar, for that matter. The science is unclear about artificial sweeteners, but my gut is telling me the we should avoid them.

Preservatives are the most harmful thing for your gut health. Think about it, what do preservatives do? They prevent organisms from digesting the product. This is all wrong, the point of eating food is to digest and absorb the nutrients. There are no organic nutrients in these products and there are also chemicals that stop the breakdown of the foods, this can cause havoc on your gut microbiome and be a major contributing factor to IBS in the first place.

If all that is not bad enough these food products are devoid of water which causes more stress on your digestive tract by pulling moisture from it and making it work harder.

"Eat whole foods in their natural form and avoid ultra-processed foods as much as possible."

Two: Fats

During a major IBS flare-up, avoiding fat is beneficial because high-fat foods can exacerbate symptoms such as bloating, gas, and abdominal pain. Fat is more challenging to digest than other macronutrients, which can slow the digestive process and increase gastrointestinal discomfort. Additionally, fats can stimulate the intestines to contract more, potentially leading to cramping and diarrhea. By avoiding high-fat foods, individuals with IBS can help reduce these symptoms and maintain better digestive health during flare ups.

Fat is an essential macronutrient and should only be avoided for a short period of time. When you are ready to start reintroducing fat, stick with animal fats as they taste great, are packed with nutrients, and are a valuable resource from the butchering process.

It's important to note that fat is where toxic chemicals are stored in the body, so try to get your animal fats from naturally raised animals as much as possible.

Recommended Animal Fats (to use after the storm has passed):

✓ Butter

✓ Lard

✓ Tallow

No matter what stage of IBS you are in, I would highly recommend never ingesting ultra-processed seed and vegetable oils. They were originally invented as industrial lubricants and these oils are highly oxidative and cause inflammation and damage cells in our bodies and block the signals from your stomach to your brain that let you know you are full.

Examples of ultra-processed seed and vegetable oils:

- Canola
- Corn
- Cottonseed
- Peanut
- Safflower
- Sesame
- Soybean
- Sunflower

Extremely high temperatures, solvents, bleach, and other harsh chemical processes are used in the refining process of these rancid oils to make them edible.

Hydrogenated oils have been chemically altered to add an extra hydrogen atom to make them solid at room temperature, used in products like margarine, Crisco, and a whole host of other processed junk food like cakes and cookies, to make them moist. They are commonly used in processed foods, fast food, and restaurants due to their affordability, availability, and high smoke point. These oils can reduce your ability to absorb nutrients and they should be avoided at all costs.

The issue is that these oils have an unhealthy balance of omega-3 and omega-6 fatty acids. In the past, we used oils with a 1:1 ratio of these fatty acids, like animal fats, but these ultra-processed oils have a 20:1 ratio of omega-6 relative to omega-3. Scientists hypothesize that eating a diet high in these oils is an underlying factor in all autoimmune diseases, heart disease, cancer, diabetes, premature aging, and arthritis.

Three: Sweeteners

Sugar is a fantastic preservative and the effect it has on your gut flora is devastating. Natural sweeteners are calorie dense and lacking in nutrients. This means you can get a lot of energy from it, but not much else.

Natural Sweeteners Include:

- Cane sugar

- Honey

- Agave Nectar

- High Fructose Corn Syrup

- Malt Extract

- Molasses

"We naturally crave sweets, but our bodies do not require them."

Artificial sweeteners can be a good tool for consuming less calories, but they are not a long-term solution. Even though they do not spike your insulin levels they can still contribute to cravings for sweets, have been shown to alter neurotransmitter levels, and are not good for your gut flora.

Artificial Sweeteners:

- Isomalt

- Maltitol

- Mannitol

- Sorbitol

- Xylitol

- Aspartame

Most of us consume more sweeteners than we should, and this is a contributing factor to many preventable diseases and especially IBS flare ups.

Don't mess around, cut out all sweeteners if you truly want to heal your gut.

Four: High Fructose Fruits

A common theme appears here and it's all about sugar. Fruits high in fructose should not be eaten during a flare up to avoid that dreaded fermentation in the large intestine that causes us so much trouble.

*"Natural and artificial
sweeteners cause problems
in your gut and beyond."*

High Fructose Fruits Include:

- Apples
- Apricots
- Blackberries
- Blueberries
- Boysenberries
- Cherries
- Dates
- Figs
- Grapes
- Nectarine
- Nectarines
- Peaches
- Pears
- Plums
- Raspberries
- Watermelon

Once your gut has settled, you can try reintroducing small amounts of these fruits back into your diet. They are a great source of fiber, vitamins and carbohydrates, especially when eaten fresh.

Five: Certain Vegetables

Vegetables high in FODMAPs are another player in the, "Will this, hurt my stomach?" game. You know what FODMAPs are by now so I'm going to list some common vegetables that are high in them, so you know not to eat them if you're in the middle of a flare up.

High FODMAP Vegetables:

- Artichokes
- Asparagus
- Beets
- Broccoli
- Brussels Sprouts
- Butternut Squash
- Cabbage
- Cauliflower
- Chile Peppers
- Corn
- Eggplant
- Fennel
- Garlic
- Leeks
- Mushrooms
- Okra
- Onions
- Peas
- Potatoes
- Shallots
- Tomatoes

Six: Lactose

All dairy contains lactose and it's one of those pesky disaccharides. So, it is in your best interest to avoid all dairy products when you're in the middle of an episode. When your gut starts to calm, you can start to reintroduce hard cheeses like cheddar, parmesan or Swiss, if you desire. These types of hard cheeses have been aged for months or even years, allowing the lactose to be converted to simpler sugars like glucose and galactose, which are mostly converted to lactic acid making these kinds of cheeses easier for your digestive system to process.

Examples of Food Containing Lactose:

- Ice Cream
- Milk
- Most Yogurts
- Soft And Fresh Cheeses (Mozzarella, Cottage Cheese, Ricotta.)
- Sour Cream
- Whey Protein Powder

Seven: Legumes

Legumes and beans are often called the "musical fruit" because they contain oligosaccharides which are hard to digest and create a lot of gas. If you eat them, they will exacerbate your symptoms.

Common Legumes Include:

- Baked Beans
- Black-Eyed Peas
- Chickpeas
- Kidney Beans
- Pinto Beans
- Soybeans
- Black Beans
- Broad Beans
- Fava Beans
- Lentils
- Red Beans
- Split Peas

Eight: Grains

Most grains are high in FODMAPs and glyphosate, a synthetic nonselective herbicide, the main ingredient in Roundup. It's found in all non-organic grains and this stuff is extremely hazardous to your gut microbiome.

The FDA found glyphosate in over 60 percent of corn and soy samples that were tested in the United States. The Environmental Working Group analyzed twenty-eight children's cereal products and found glyphosate in all of them!

A German study took urine samples from 140 subjects and found glyphosate in all samples but showed a significantly lower amount in those who self-reported eating an organic diet.

If you can afford organic grain products, I highly recommend you buy them when you are ready to reintroduce grains back into your diet.

Glyphosate is thought to cause cancer and has been shown to have detrimental health effects on the gut microbiome and the microbiome of the soil, which we rely on to feed the crops we depend on.

If FODMAPs and glyphosate weren't bad enough grains like wheat, barley, and rye also contain gluten. The genetically modified wheat we have in the United States has much more gluten than heritage wheat, and it causes inflammation in the digestive system. Gluten isn't a known trigger of IBS but it's not helping. You may not be particularly sensitive to gluten, as far as you know. An elimination diet is the best way to find out. Either way, limiting foods like breads and pastas made with wheat will make a big impact on improving your health.

Grains high in FODMAPS:

- Barley
  - Beer
  - Whisky
- Corn
  - Breakfast Cereals
  - Chips
  - Tortillas
- Rye
  - Pumpernickel
- Wheat
  - Biscuits
  - Bread
  - Breakfast Cereals
  - Crackers
  - Pancakes
  - Pasta
  - Tortillas
  - Waffles

Nine: Certain Beverages

Not drinking certain beverages when you're in the middle of an IBS attack can make a huge impact on whether your gut starts healing or gets worse. You may have never considered that some beverages could be causing you issues, especially coconut water due to the fermentable sugars it contains!

Beverages to Avoid:

Alcohol: Alcohol irritates the gut lining, disrupts the gut microbiota, and worsens IBS symptoms.

Fortified Wines: High in sugars and alcohol, both of which can irritate the gut and disrupt normal digestive function.

Fruit Juices: Often high in fructose, a type of sugar that is poorly absorbed in the small intestine and can lead to bloating and diarrhea.

Oat and Soy Milk: This milk alternative is high in FODMAPs due to the presence of oligosaccharides. Some oat milks contains added sugars and thickeners that are problematic.

Soft Drinks with High Fructose Corn Syrup: Obviously high in fructose and highly processed, these drinks can cause digestive issues and trigger IBS symptoms.

Tea (Chai, Chamomile, Fennel): While not all teas are problematic, these specific types can contain compounds that may stimulate the gut or cause allergic reactions. For example, chai often contains caffeine and spices, chamomile can cause allergic reactions in some people, and fennel can have a laxative effect.

Avoiding these drinks during an IBS attack can help manage symptoms and promote better gut health.

Ten: Eggs

Eggs are one of the healthiest foods you can eat as they are full of protein, fat, and many micronutrients. Sadly, when you're in the middle of the storm, it might be a good idea to cut them out of your diet until the storm passes.

Eggs are the only food on the list that do not contain FODMAPS. However, they do contain sulfur, which may exacerbate bloating, and excessive gas.

Some readers may also be sensitive to eggs, whether it be due to the corn and soy feeds used in commercial egg laying operations, or the herbicides and pesticides used to grow those feeds. The management practices of the operation itself, the lack of a natural diet, or any hormones and antibiotics given to the layers.

Then there is the fat component. Those who are suffering with IBS-D may feel the effects of eating high fat foods more than others, because fat increases gut motility, which moves foods through your gut more quickly leading to, you guessed it, diarrhea.

Chapter Summary:

That's it for the top ten foods to avoid, but I would also strongly encourage you to stay away from smoking, and vaping, as these activities can also exacerbate IBS symptoms.

It may be hard at first to adapt to a new way of eating but once you start to feel better you will know it was worth it. Remember the first few weeks will be the hardest but once you are able to stop eating the foods that are hurting you, the craving for those foods starts to go away and your body will start to crave the foods that nourish it.

In "The Dorito Effect", Mark Schatzker goes into great detail on this subject and explains how processed foods hijack our natural ability to crave the food that contain the specific nutrients our bodies need by using artificial flavors and calorie rich, nutrient poor food products.

The good news is that you will not have to avoid these foods for the rest of your life, but you will have to wait to eat them again until your gut is healed and then and only then can you slowly start incorporating very small amounts of these foods into your diet again.

"Let food be thy medicine and medicine be thy food."

-Hippocrates

CHAPTER 6:
TOP TEN FOODS TO INCLUDE:
TO PREVENT AN IBS ATTACK

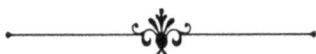

Six weeks after John tried the bone broth fast, he was feeling like his old self again. He only consumed bone broth and water that first week, allowing his gut time to start repairing itself and begin the healing process. After that first week, he continued drinking bone broth every day, and he also started incorporating lean meats and eggs back into his diet.

John was feeling good, but he was scared that if he ate the wrong thing, he would have another episode. This is normal, but it is important to start reintroducing other foods so you can get a well-rounded diet and truly know what specific foods trigger you. John discovered the foods that triggered him by doing an elimination diet and then adding the foods mentioned in this chapter into his diet first. He did this one at a time and in small amounts in case one of them had a bad reaction in his gut.

This is a classic example of how you can take your health back by changing what you eat. An elimination diet may not be easy to stick to, but neither is daily suffering. If you can stick with it for long enough, your digestive system will thank you and you will have more autonomy. Once your gut is healed from a specific flare up you should continue to avoid the foods listed in Chapter 5 as much as possible and include the foods that will prevent future attacks.

THE TOP TEN FOODS TO INCLUDE:

1. Bone Broth
2. Fermented Foods
3. Animal Protein
4. High Fiber Foods
5. Eggs
6. Organic Fruits
7. Whole Raw Dairy Products
8. Ginger
9. Rice
10. No Food

One: Bone Broth

Liquid gold, also known as bone broth, is a nutritious liquid made by boiling bones and the connective tissues of animals. It has a long history across different cultures around the world. Its roots can be traced back to prehistoric times when no part of the animal was wasted. These broths are easy to make and should be made at home for the best results.

Bone broth contains collagen and gelatin, which can help support and repair the intestinal lining. This is crucial for IBS sufferers who may have a compromised gut barrier. It's also a good source of minerals like calcium, magnesium, and phosphorus, which are essential for overall health but are particularly important for maintaining digestive health. Compared to other foods that might trigger IBS symptoms, bone broth is easy to digest and low in FODMAPs. You will need to remove the fat from bone broth for the first few days as it can be hard to digest.

If providing essential nutrients, soothing, and healing your gut weren't enough to sell you on how awesome bone broth is, it also provides hydration.

Bone broth is great on its own or can be used as an ingredient in many recipes. You can substitute it for water when steaming rice or use it as a base to make soup. Some components in bone broth, like glycine, are thought to have anti-inflammatory properties.

I recommend you make bone broth yourself, as the store bought broths just do not compare to the nutrient density of a homemade broth, there are also preservatives and other undesirable ingredients used in store bought broth, they are okay in a pinch, but if you want the full effect you are going to have to make it yourself or find local sources of fresh or frozen bone broth. In the next chapter, I will teach you how you can make it at home with just a few simple ingredient.

Two: Fermented foods

Every traditional culture around the world has at least one fermented food or beverage as a staple in their diet. Kimchi in Korea, Kombucha in China, and Sauerkraut in Germany.

We have Lactobacillus, a genius of bacteria to thank for transforming these foods into super foods. When the lactobacillus bacteria start to break down the carbohydrates like glucose, fructose, and lactose, lactic acid is produced and provides a natural preservative and gives these fermented foods their sour taste. It also promotes the growth of good microbes in your intestines, provides pH balance, and is antimicrobial which helps fight infections.

The fermentation process makes the nutrients in the foods more bioavailable so we can get the maximum benefit of eating these foods and the best part is all these microbes are probiotic which support gut health, improve digestion, strengthen the immune system, and can even improve mental health!

Some studies suggest that the consumption of certain fermented foods can reduce the risk of chronic diseases such as heart disease, diabetes, and cancer. This could be due to the reduction of anti-nutrients and the production of beneficial metabolites like certain fatty acids and antioxidants during fermentation.

Common Fermented Foods:

- ✓ Kimchi (Korea)
- ✓ Beet Kvass (Russia)
- ✓ Kombucha (China)
- ✓ Tempeh (Indonesia)
- ✓ Sauerkraut (Germany)
- ✓ Kefir (Eastern Europe)
- ✓ Miso (Japan)
- ✓ Yogurt (Middle East)
- ✓ Pickled Vegetables (Ancient Egypt)
- ✓ Ginger bug soda (Unknown Origin)

As usual, I recommend you make your own fermented foods or purchase them from a trusted source. Pickles you buy in the store are not fermented, they are pickled in vinegar and do not offer the same probiotic benefits as fermented foods.

Three: Animal Protein

Most people do not eat enough protein. Trust me, I know, I wrote a whole book about it called *Living The Protein Lifestyle*. Plant proteins just can't compete with the nutrient density, bioavailability, and its amino acid profile.

Eating more meat is not only going to provide you with the vital macronutrients your body needs but it will keep you feeling full and power you through your day. If your gut is still sensitive from a flare up, stick with lean meats like chicken breast or top sirloin steak.

Fat, including cholesterol, is a vital component of all of the cells in your body, especially your brain. Seventy-five percent of your brain is made of myelin and myelin is made from cholesterol. It's also a key component in making vitamin D which is critical for hormone production. So, make sure to add fat back into your diet when you can.

Suggested Animal Proteins:

- ✓ Beef
- ✓ Lamb
- ✓ Pork
- ✓ Chicken
- ✓ Turkey
- ✓ Organ Meats

Meat from naturally raised animals is always best and can be bought directly from local producers, subscription box services, or from animal share programs. It's best to support local ranchers if possible as they produce the healthiest animals and they need your help to compete with the mega corporations.

Check out eatwild.com to find locally Produced Animal Protein (Click "Shop for Local Grassfed Meat, Eggs & Dairy")

"Animal protein is the most nutrient dense and bioavailable food on the planet."

Four: High Fiber Foods

Fiber is a tricky for those with IBS. It's vital to feed your gut flora but can also cause problems with fermentation in your gut. This is why you should wait until your symptoms have diminished and your gut has healed before you start adding fiber back to your diet.

When your digestive system is able to handle some FODMAPs again make sure to include foods high in fiber back into your diet. There are two types of fiber: soluble and insoluble.

Soluble fiber dissolves in water and forms a gel like substance in your gut slowing down digestion and allowing for better absorption of nutrients and reducing blood sugar spikes. It also feeds your gut flora, but this can be problematic because to feed your gut flora the soluble fiber is fermented in your large intestine and when this process gets out of control it is one of the major causes of IBS symptoms.

Insoluble fiber does not break down in water, adding bulk to your stool which helps keep your bowel movements regular. It can also make symptoms worse so be careful and take it slow with insoluble fiber.

Recommended High Fiber foods:

- ✓ Fruits:
  - o Blueberries
  - o Strawberries
  - o Raspberries
- ✓ Vegetables:
  - o Carrots
  - o Eggplant
  - o Zucchini
- ✓ Nuts and Seeds
  - o Almonds
  - o Pumpkin seeds
  - o Chia seeds
- ✓ Grains
  - o Quinoa
  - o Oats
  - o Brown rice
- ✓ Psyllium husk

Five: Eggs

These oval wonders are the only items on both the foods to avoid and the foods to include lists. They can be problematic during a flare up due to their high fat content, but if you are not sensitive or allergic to eggs then you should definitely be eating them on a regular basis once your gut has calmed down.

The best eggs are from backyard producers who free range their chickens. These chickens get the sunlight, fresh air, and nutrients they need to produce nutrient dense eggs. They eat a more natural diet than their factory farmed brethren and may even get to eat a bug or two providing all kinds of good nutrition.

If you can't get fresh eggs try to buy organic pasture raised eggs, They are packed with tons of minerals and vitamins, plus protein, and that wonderful cholesterol your body needs to function properly.

Six: Organic Fruits

Eating organic fruit will add fiber to your diet and can satisfy your sweet tooth while still avoiding those pesky ultra-processed food products. If you stick with low fructose fruits, it will help keep your gut in check and prevent future attacks. When you spend that extra money to buy organic fruit you get the added benefit of knowing that it was not sprayed with glyphosate.

I love papaya, because it tastes like candy and contains papain, a proteolytic enzyme that helps with digestion. If you pair papaya with banana, it's transformative. Stick with semi-green bananas, they offer more fiber and less sugar.

Recommended Low Fructose Fruits:

- ✓ Banana
- ✓ Blueberry
- ✓ Cantaloupe
- ✓ Cranberry
- ✓ Grape
- ✓ Kiwi
- ✓ Lemon
- ✓ Lime
- ✓ Orange
- ✓ Papaya
- ✓ Strawberry

Seven: Whole Raw Dairy Products

Whole raw milk has the essential fats we need along with enzymes that will aid your digestion. If your tummy can't handle cow's milk, try drinking goat's milk. The fat globules are smaller and easier to digest. I would highly recommend not drinking nut "milks," as they can cause a plethora of gut issues due to how they are processed and they do not provide a lot of nutrients.

On the other hand, milk from grass fed cows can aid in digestion, support immune system function, provide probiotics, and it tastes good.

You can also make cheese, yogurt, butter, and kefir from raw milk if pure milk is too much for your gut. If you do make cheese save the whey and use it to boost your fermented vegetables or drink a shot a day to help you stay strong and healthy.

If you are sensitive to dairy or still avoiding fermentable sugars stick with low lactose cheeses that may be better tolerated.

"Whole raw milk is a super food!"

Low Lactose cheeses:

Type of Cheese	Lactose per 100g	Recommended Serving Size
Blue Cheese	0 – 0.5	40g
Camembert Cheese	0.1g – 0.46	40g
Cheddar Cheese	0.1g – 0.48	40g
Cheshire Cheese	0.0g	40g
Brie & Camembert	0.1g – 0.46g	40g
Colby Cheese	0.1g – 0.69g	40g
Creamed Cottage Cheese	1.9g – 2.67g	40g
Feta Cheese	0.1g to 4.09	40g
Pecorino Style Cheese	0.2g	40g
Swiss Cheese	0.0g – 0.1g	40g
Havarti	0.1g	40g
Monterey Jack	0.1g	40g
Manchego Cheese	0.1g	40g
Mozzarella Cheese	0.1g – 1.0g	40g
Parmesan	0.0 – 0.07	40g.

Eight: Ginger

The root of the ginger plant has a calming effect on the digestive tract, it reduces gastrointestinal irritation, suppresses gastric contractions or stomach cramps, and alleviates bloating and gas. It's great for reducing nausea and has anti-inflammatory and antioxidant properties.

Ginger can enhance digestion by stimulating the production of digestive enzymes, which can help ease symptoms of IBS.

Because of all of these benefits I have included ginger in my bone broth recipe in Chapter 7. Ginger can also be consumed in a pill, as a tea, or used to flavor foods. I recommend you consume ginger in its natural whole food form for best results, for example you can use fresh ginger root to make a simple tea.

Drinking ginger tea to calm an upset stomach can help tremendously and it can avoid further irritation which left untreated could contribute to an IBS flare up.

Nine: Rice

Rice is inexpensive and widely available. Brown rice (whole grain rice) seems to be tolerated by some, while white rice seems to be tolerated by almost everyone. From my research, the bran in brown rice may be a trigger for some, so if that's you, stick to white rice.

I recommend purchasing rice that has no additives and is not enriched like Mahatma or Uncle Bens, as the synthetic vitamins and minerals used to enrich the rice may trigger symptoms. I love jasmine rice, but basmati or plain old long grain rice is good too.

Short grain rice on the other hand, is absorbed faster in your gut causing insulin spikes and could cause gut motility issues leading to a flare up, so stick with long grain rice and if you can tolerate it, make it brown rice.

If you want to do your gut a favor, try soaking your rice in water. You can do this for one hour or up to 12 hours. This will allow enzymes to start breaking down the starches, making the final product easier to digest.

Ten: No Food

Okay you got me, the last item on the list is not a food, it's the lack of food and most beverages for a short time compared to traditional fasting. Intermittent fasting is a fantastic way to give your gut a break and let it clear out all the food you ate and allow it to start settling down. Fasting may be scary to some, but you actually do it every night when you sleep. That is why we call it breakfast, you are literally breaking your overnight fast when you eat that first meal of the day.

If you put in a little effort, you can extend your nightly fast easily and reap the rewards. For example, if you stop eating at 8pm and then wait to eat breakfast until 8am, you just did a twelve hour fast and that is a great starting point. From there you can extend it further by skipping breakfast and eating lunch at noon. Bam! You just did a sixteen hour fast. This will trigger autophagy, that's when your body starts to clear out dead or damaged cells and even uses the components of some of those old cells to repair others. This is also when your liver gets time to clear out the extra fat stored there and do some repairs.

You can cheat a little by drinking some black coffee or plain tea if the caffeine doesn't bother you. When you start to really feel hungry try drinking water to fill your belly, it helps more than you would think. Once you get past the nauseous stage, you'll be home free and may be able to go all day without eating...

It's challenging to start fasting but once you are successful at it you could become addicted. When you are intermittent fasting, you must make sure you are eating enough because it's a form of calorie restriction. If you don't consume your recommended allotment your body could start to slow down your metabolism to preserve the calories you do eat, this is all bad for IBS and for weight management. Eat enough food so your body has the energy to get you through your day and repair itself.

Chapter Summary

John was able to find foods that did not mess him up and you can too. It's not easy but it is possible to overcome IBS and get your life back. You must track what you eat, how it affects you, and your bowel movements to figure out what foods are triggering your symptoms. Pretend you are a detective and you're trying to solve a mystery. The mystery of what made my stomach hurt today. It's too hard to remember how you felt, everything you ate, drank, and every bowel movement, but if you take notes, you can go back and figure out what triggered you.

Over time certain foods may start to bother you and the reverse is also true. You may be able to eat some foods in the future that you can't eat now. So, make sure to keep a positive mindset and continue to experiment by trying different foods from time to time, in small amounts at first and in close proximity to a toilet. Just in case.

CHAPTER 7:
FIVE RECIPES FOR RELIEF:
From A Major Flare Up

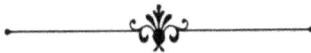

C ooking your own food is the only way to be sure of what is in it and the manner of preparation. If you go out to eat at a restaurant and you want to know about a particular item on the menu, you could ask the waiter. They may not know or they may tell you what they think is in it, or they'll tell you what they think you want to hear. This is not going to help you with your IBS because you are not in control of the ingredients or the process and that's what is required to get through an attack.

When you cook your own food, you get to choose every aspect of how it's prepared, and you'll be better able to identify and avoid your triggers. If you're in the middle of a flare up, make your food as bland as possible. Herbs and spices used to flavor foods may be triggering you and should be avoided until your gut has calmed down.

Without further ado, here are the top five recipes for IBS relief.

One: Chicken Bone Broth

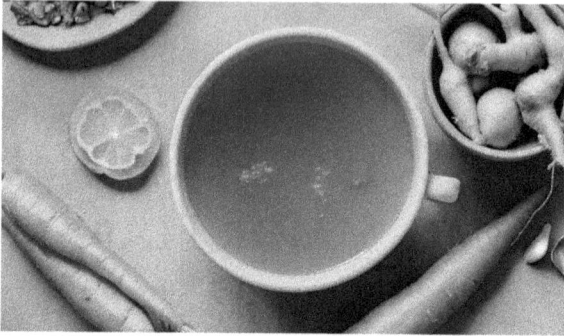

You know the benefits of drinking bone broth from the previous chapters and now I will teach you how to make your own. This is a great recipe for all IBS types, and it can also help if you have a cold or flu. It's a simple yet powerful recipe to reduce irritation in your stomach, the ginger helps calm the stomach and the collagen and gelatin will repair it. If you make this right, the whole thing should firm up like Jell-O, after refrigeration. That is a sign that there is enough collagen and gelatin, and that will do a lot for the health of your gut mucosa, skin, hair, and joints!

This chicken bone broth recipe is easy to make and digest. The ginger will calm your stomach and relieve many IBS symptoms. You can make a beef version of this recipe if you substitute the chicken legs for beef shanks and once the IBS storm has passed you can add all kinds of additional ingredients to make this broth more flavorful like garlic and onions.

This broth can be drunk on its own or used as an ingredient in many recipes. You can use it to steam rice to add flavor and additional nutrients or use it as a stock for soups and stews. It is very versatile and can be stored in the freezer for many months.

Ingredients:

3-4 quarts of filtered water

4 lbs. of chicken legs

3 large carrots washed, ends cut off, and rough chopped.

2 inches ginger washed and roughly chopped.

1 medium lemon, zested and juice lemon only

1 bunch cilantro stems, washed and stems chopped off, use leaves for another dish.

2 tablespoons apple cider vinegar

2 teaspoons salt

Directions:

1. Combine ingredients into a large stock pot or a 6 quart or larger pressure cooker like an instant pot.

2. Cook the broth:

   a) Pressure cooker: Seal and pressure cook on high for 2 hours and let it naturally release the pressure for at least 20 minutes.

   b) Stock Pot: Cook over high heat until it boils then reduce to medium heat, cover, and let simmer for 4-8 hours.

3. Once cooled, strain broth with a metal colander, discard or feed the meat and carrots to your dogs, and let the broth cool in the refrigerator overnight.

4. Finish by scraping the fat off of the top (If you're not in a flare up keep the fat).

5. The broth can be stored in your refrigerator for up to 1 week or in your freezer for up to 3 months.

Two: Steamed Rice +

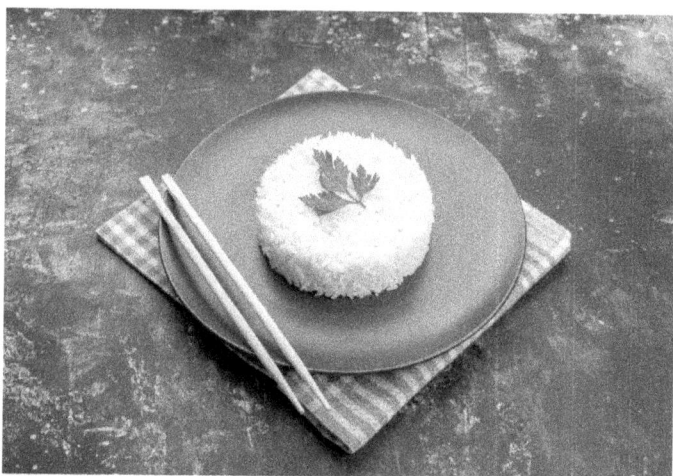

Steamed white rice is a great source of calories and easy to digest especially if you soak the rice before you cook it. Soaking allows the enzymes to start breaking down the starches making it easy for your body to get as much of the nutrition from it as possible and reducing stress on your digestive system at the same time. Keep in mind the longer you soak your rice the less time it will need to cook.

Making the perfect steamed rice can be tricky and the recipe may need some adjustment depending on your situation but once you get the timing down it will come out perfect every time. The type of equipment, type of rice, and even your elevation can change cooking times and the quantity of the cooking liquid can be the difference between mushy or fluffy rice. If it comes out mushy, try reducing the amount of cooking liquid; if it's chewy or undercooked, try adding a tad more cooking liquid and cook it a little longer.

Ingredients:

2 cups of rice, rinse rice and soak for at least one hour, strain and rinse one more time.
3 cups of chicken bone broth, fat removed

Directions:
Rice cooker:

1. Put the bone broth into the rice cooker pot.
2. Add the rice and stir.
3. Push the start button and wait until it's done cooking.
4. Fluff with a fork and enjoy.

Pressure cooker:

1. Put the bone broth into the pressure cooker pot.
2. Add the rice and stir.
3. Seal and cook on high pressure for 4 minutes and let the pressure naturally release for 10 minutes.
4. Fluff with a fork and enjoy.

Saucepan:

1. Put the bone broth into the saucepan.
2. Set over high heat until it starts to boil.
3. Add the rice and stir.
4. Cover the pot, reduce to medium heat, and let simmer for about 18 minutes.
5. Remove from heat, leave lid on the saucepan, and allow the rice to steam for 5 minutes.
6. Fluff with a fork and enjoy.

Three: Simple Ground Beef

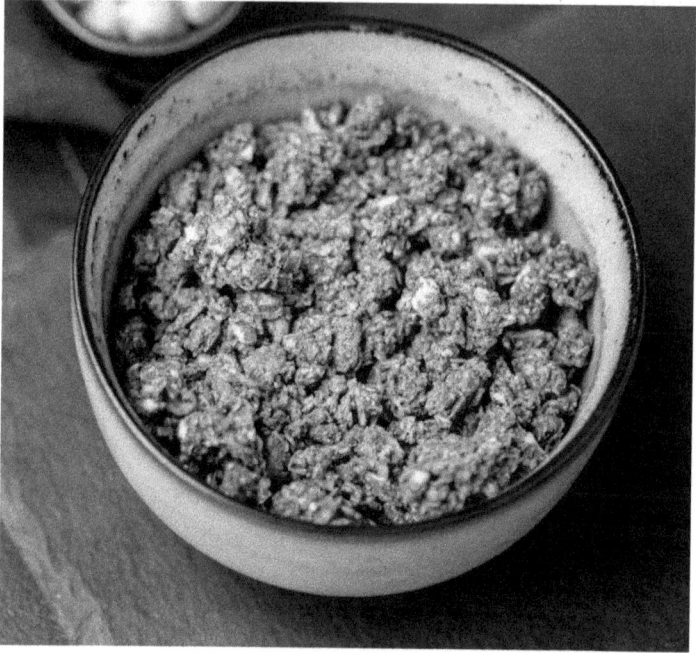

This ground beef recipe is simple and easy to make. It is very basic but will provide you with the vital protein and micronutrients your body needs to feel better. You can substitute the ground beef in the recipe with ground chicken or turkey if that suits you better, but beef is the best by far due to its nutritional profile.

Ingredients:
1 pound of lean ground beef
1 teaspoon of salt

Directions:

1. Place a skillet over medium heat.

2. Add the ground beef, break it up using a spatula, and distribute across the pan evenly.

3. Add the salt and continue breaking up the ground beef and mixing with a spatula.

4. Mix and flip the ground beef every few minutes until fully cooked.

5. Strain out any leftover grease in the pan using a metal colander.

Ginger Bug Soda

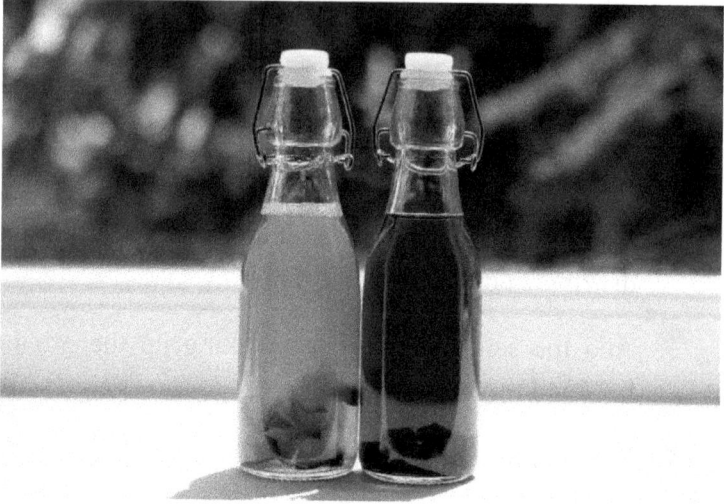

Homemade soft drinks are a fantastic way to give yourself a special treat and get your daily dose of probiotics at the same time. The magic comes from natural bacteria found on the ginger and native yeasts in your home. When you submerge the ginger under water it creates an aerobic environment where culture starts to grow and when you feed it sugar this process goes into overdrive.

Key factors for success:

- The water must be filtered to avoid chlorine which can affect fermentation.

- You need to use a caloric sweetener like sugar to feed your bug, stevia or other non-caloric sweeteners will not work.

  o White sugar works best but you could try using honey or molasses for a different flavor profile.

- Keep the ginger bug away from other cultures like sauerkraut and kombucha or it could cross culture and ruin the batch.

There is some debate about whether it is better to peel the root or not. My general rule is that non-organic ginger gets peeled and organic is only rinsed before grating. If you don't have a greater, you can finely chop the ginger instead of grating it.

Once the ginger bug has cultured, it can be used at the ratio of ¼ cup ginger bug starter per quart of sweetened herbal mixtures (for ginger ale or root beer) or diluted fruit juice to create fruit flavored sodas.

The longer you ferment your beverages, the more sugar will be consumed by the microbes and the beverage will become more carbonated and slightly alcoholic so be careful.

Ginger Bug:

The Ginger Bug is a mixture of ginger, sugar, and water. As it ferments it releases carbon dioxide (CO_2) which is what carbonates the soda. It's what was used to make natural sodas like old fashioned ginger ale or root beer back in the day and it's a great way to repopulate your gut microbiome with beneficial microbes.

ingredients:
2-3 tablespoons (1.5-2 inches) of ginger root, washed and grated.
2-3 tablespoons white sugar
2 cups filtered water

Directions:

1. Place an equal amount of ginger and white sugar in a quart size mason jar.

2. Add the filtered water to the Mason jar.

3. Stir with a non-metal spoon and cover with a coffee filter and rubber band so it can breathe.

4. Every day for the next five days, stir the mixture at least once and add 1 tablespoon of grated ginger and 1 tablespoon of sugar.

5. Depending on temperature, it may take four to eight days to create the bug.

6. You can tell if your ginger bug is ready if there are bubbles forming around the top of the mixture, and it "fizzes" when stirred, and it takes on a sweet and mildly yeasty smell.

7. It should become somewhat cloudy and opaque.

8. If mold appears on the top, scrape it off if it can be removed. If this happens more than once, you will need to start again.

9. If the mixture hasn't taken on these characteristics by the 7th or 8th day, you need to discard it and start again.

10. Try using a glass fermentation weight to hold the ginger down under the surface of the water. This is an anaerobic process, so keeping the mixture submerged is required for proper fermentation.

11. To keep your ginger bug alive, you will need to feed it regularly.

12. Add 1 teaspoon of minced ginger and 1 teaspoon of sugar per day if kept at room temperature.

13. You can also "rest" it in the fridge and feed it 1 tablespoon each of ginger and sugar once a week.

14. To reactivate your ginger bug remove it from the fridge, let it reach room temperature and begin feeding it again daily.

Homemade Natural Sodas:

Ingredients:

¼ cup of ginger bug

1 quart of (low FODMAP) fresh fruit juice

Directions:

1. Strain your ginger bug.

2. Add your fruit juice and mix well.

3. Pour the mixture into swing top bottles, mason jars, or another vessel that will hold some pressure.

4. Seal your vessels and let sit out for 3-5 days.

5. Test your soda by opening a vessel (Over the sink) to see how carbonated it is.

   1. If you like it, transfer your sodas to the fridge to stop the fermentation process.

   2. If you want it more carbonated and less sweet let it sit out another day or so.

Natural Soda Flavor Ideas:

- ✓ Apple
- ✓ Lemon
- ✓ Lime
- ✓ Papaya

Five: Fermented Vegetables

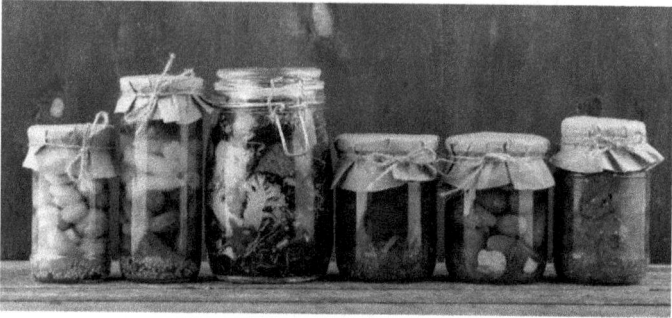

I will offer several fermented vegetable options and share one recipe with you that I eat as a garnish almost every day to keep my gut in tip top shape.

There are so many options for fermented vegetables, if you don't like one, keep experimenting until you find one you love. You can also play with how long you ferment different vegetables to discover your preferences.

The process of fermentation is the same for most vegetables. You either draw out the liquid from the vegetable itself or you use a saltwater brine. Like the ginger bug you will need to keep the oxygen away from the vegetables by keeping them submerged under the brine so the microbes can go to work.

Recommended Vegetables for Fermentation:

- ✓ Beets
- ✓ Cabbage (Sauerkraut)
- ✓ Carrots
- ✓ Cucumbers (Real Pickles)
- ✓ Daikon Radish
- ✓ Napa Cabbage (Kimchee)

Probiotic Carrot Sticks
Ingredients:

- 3 cups of filtered water

- 2 pounds carrots, washed, peel, and cut into sticks

- 1 1/2 tablespoons of kosher salt

Directions:

1. Combine the water and the salt and stir until the salt is fully dissolved to create the brine.

2. Pack your carrots tightly into a mason jar or other container so that they stay submerged once the brine is added.

    1. You may need to use a glass fermentation weight to keep them submerged.

3. Cover carrots with your saltwater brine.

4. Leave your carrots on the counter overnight or up to a week depending on the temperature and how fermented you like your carrots.

5. Put them in the fridge to stop the fermentation process.

6. Enjoy a few fermented carrot sticks with each meal to aid in digestion.

Check out ww.nourishedkitchen.com for more fermented food and drink recipes.

Chapter Summary:

The best tip I can give you to help with your IBS and overall health is to cook as much of the food you eat as possible. There are so many cumulative benefits to cooking your own food that it can make a huge impact on your overall health.

It takes time to cook and prepare food to eat so if you're not hungry you will be less likely to snack if you have to go out of your way to prepare something. It also helps avoid binge eating, especially if you only prepare enough for one snack. You are also in control of every aspect of your meal, what kind of oil you cook with and how much or what kind of seasoning you use (lots of them have sugar). These small details can add up and make a big difference in how you will feel after eating.

Saving money is an added bonus. It may seem expensive when you buy groceries but if you consider how much food you can make compared to how much you can buy for the same amount, it's the obvious choice. Also, if you save your scraps, you can make broths and soups for pennies.

I suggest you try one new recipe a week to build a solid foundation of recipes you can rely on, ones that you know how to make and enjoy. If you don't like a particular recipe, modify it or never make it again. The most important part of cooking is that you are in the driver's seat and you can customize recipes to fit your tastes. Add or remove ingredients as needed and make it your own. If you don't have an ingredient, use a substitute or skip it all together if appropriate.

Cooking can be fun and rewarding so give these recipes a shot and see how they make you feel after you eat them. I bet you'll feel great!

CHAPTER 8:
STRESS AND IBS:
GET YOUR MIND RIGHT

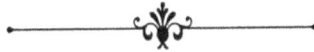

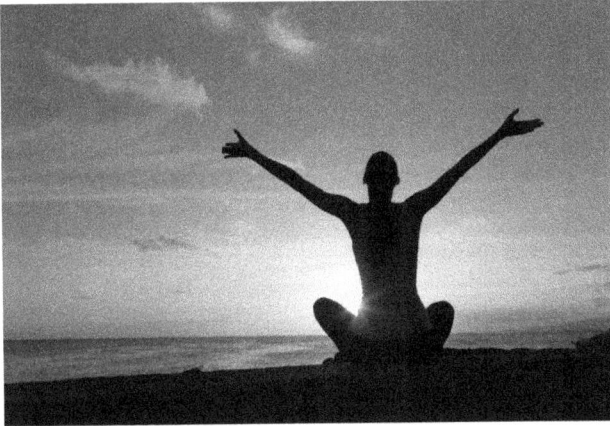

All the guys were outside the bathroom, banging on the door. "I got to go man, get out of there!" One of them said.

They probably think I'm masturbating in here, but that's better than them knowing the truth. Bill thought.

Bill was a firefighter, and he was still dealing with bouts of constipation. He had been on the toilet so long his feet were numb, and his firefighting companions didn't know what was taking him so long. Bill was ashamed and didn't want to tell them what was going on with him.

One day Bill saw a reel online about how stress can have a severe impact on gut health and he wondered if that could be the root cause of his troubles. He had tried an elimination diet, but he could not stick with it and after his little episode in the gym, he never went anywhere without his water bottle and electrolytes.

He thought about how he could reduce stress at work. *What do I have to lose? I've tried everything else.*

He told Sylvia, his girlfriend, his theory about the link between his stress at work and his IBS, but she was not very supportive. Bill spent a lot of time at the firehouse and thought that maybe the guys would understand or at least be forced by the captain or HR to comply.

The next day, Bill finally came clean and told the guys about his IBS. They were so cool about it. Johnny Blaze said, "Is that why you spend so much time in the bathroom?"

"Yes, and I think my stress is the trigger to it all." Bill said.

Everyone agreed to try to reduce the stress levels in the firehouse when they were not on an emergency call. They started meditating together every morning and practiced open communication. Bill ended up breaking up with Sylvia as she was not supportive, and she was another stressor in his life.

A few weeks later, Bill was feeling better. He was amazed that the additional stress from trying to keep his high maintenance girlfriend happy and hiding his IBS at work, really was making his IBS worse. Once the stress was gone, Bill continued to exercise, and stay hydrated, resulting in a big improvement.

Bill is an excellent example of how stress can exacerbate IBS symptoms. Your emotional state may seem trivial, but the gut brain axis is real, and your thoughts affect your gut and vice versa.

Some may try to reduce stress by emotional eating, drinking alcohol, or smoking, however these practices only make your symptoms worse. Alcohol makes you feel good in the moment, but it is a poison, and it causes chaos for your gut flora and adds an additional strain on your liver when you drink in excess. Smoking can cause inflammation and can disrupt the balance of microbes in your gut, in addition to all the other known health factors.

One of the worst feelings and greatest cause of stress is helplessness. That feeling you get when you just can't figure out what is wrong with you and you're desperate for an answer to your distress. Remember how Barbara was able to find relief by eliminating the top ten foods to avoid? Well, the real catalyst to her salvation was a diagnosis from her long-time family doctor. The simple act of receiving a diagnosis from a trusted source was what gave her the confidence that she needed to beat it.

She trusted her doctor and when she told her what was wrong, Barbara felt a sense of relief that was communicated via the vagus nerve, and it had a positive impact on her gut health. Barbara's diagnosis made all the difference and got her rolling down the path to recovery and motivated her to start making better food choices.

Solutions for Stress Reduction:

- ✓ Exercise
- ✓ Walking
- ✓ Good Sleep
- ✓ Practicing Gratitude
- ✓ Meditation
- ✓ Overcoming Challenges
- ✓ Positive Affirmations
- ✓ Spending Time in Nature
- ✓ Talking With a Qualified Mental Health Professional
- ✓ Positive Mindset

Chapter Summary:

Reducing stress will do a whole lot more than just help you recover from IBS. It can also help you live longer and give you a better quality of life. If you can learn to incorporate only a few of the solutions listed above it could be the beginning of your recovery from your tummy troubles. It's also helpful to think of IBS as something that happens to you, not something you're born with, and you have the power to fix it!

You can do this, start by taking on one new stress reduction strategy one at a time and build from there. I believe mental health is the most important factor to overall health.

CHAPTER 9:
ACTIVITY:
THE MISSING LINK

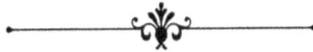

———— ⚜ ————

He glanced in her direction, she smiled, so he smiled back and continued his set of bodyweight squats.

John had gotten a membership at his local gym and had hired a trainer to show him the proper form of the exercises so he wouldn't hurt himself.

John was feeling better after he completed an elimination diet, he started adding foods back into his diet. He was a little overweight and depressed. John recently read a book that mentioned how physical activity could help with depression and weight loss, so he started working out every day at the gym and had made a friend.

John was single and he was so passionate about his job as a schoolteacher that he would regularly stay late to finish up his work, he did not have a girlfriend or much of a life outside of work.

After his surgery scare, he started looking at his life from a different perspective. He started putting his health first. After school he would go straight to the gym and get a workout in and then go home and cook dinner, then go for a nice relaxing walk. He started waking up early to cook his breakfast and go to school early to get as much work done as possible before class started.

This small change in his routine made a world of difference for John. He started talking to that cute girl he saw in the gym and now he had a date on Friday night. Things were looking up for John and he was feeling and looking better than ever.

"Small changes over time will make a big impact." Being active is beneficial for your gut, when you move your body, you help your digestive system function better. The motility of your gut can be improved by moving your body.

Walking is one of the best things you can do for your overall health and it's especially powerful when done after each meal and at a quick pace. You may be busy and find it hard to make time for this but even a short walk after each meal will do wonders for your digestion.

In my workbook *The Protein Lifestyle Workbook*, I go into great detail about the different types of exercise, including strength training, mobility practices, and cardiovascular exercise. All you need to know is that the more you move your body the better you will feel. Now, you can overdo it, so take it easy at first. If you live a sedentary lifestyle, adding some activity to your life will go a long way to relieve your gastrointestinal plight.

Some readers may be asking "What if I can't afford a gym membership?" The answer is, you don't need one, you can move your body and get some physical activity in many ways.

Low-Cost Activities:

- ✓ Bike riding
- ✓ Gardening
- ✓ Hiking
- ✓ Household Chores
- ✓ Stretching
- ✓ Swimming
- ✓ Walking
- ✓ Yoga

Chapter Summary:

The best activity you can do for your overall health is strength training. Some examples include weightlifting, resistance band training, yoga, and body weight exercises. These types of exercises help to strengthen your bones and your muscles, making you more resilient to injuries. Having more muscle can contribute to a better mental outlook as well.

Whatever you decide to do, start slow and small, so you don't hurt yourself, find something you like and do it regularly. Pick something, anything and give it a go.

This practice will contribute to much more than improving your gut health, it can make the difference between enjoying life or just existing.

CHAPTER 10:
HYDRATION:
IT'S NOT JUST ABOUT
DRINKING WATER

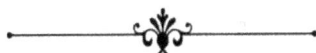

———— ⚜ ————

❝❝That dude just passed out right in the middle of his kettle bell swing!" That's what Bill heard as he came to, that day he passed out in the gym. He was so embarrassed he left the gym as fast as he could. After talking with his health coach, Bill realized that he was dehydrated, and this was contributing to his constipation and his embarrassing episode in the gym.

He was drinking water, but his super strict diet of whole foods didn't supply him with enough sodium, one of the essential electrolytes our bodies require to get water into our cells where we need it. He knew all about hydration as a firefighter but he didn't realize how little sodium he was consuming since he cooked most of his food himself and didn't add much salt.

After that day in the gym, he started adding more salt to his food and started adding electrolytes into his water when he needed more.

If you start to run low on water your body will go into survival mode and pull water in the form of blood from your organs to preserve the brain and heart. This also results in less saliva as the first step in digestion along with chewing. It is important to have properly pre-moistened food for your stomach to do its job. Reduced digestive juices in your gut will result as well and to top it all off, blood is pulled from your gut further reducing its ability to function properly. All of this will lead to hard stool and constipation.

Ways Our Bodies Loose Water:

- Breathing
- Diarrhea
- Exercising
- Sweating
- Vomiting

Staying hydrated is not only about drinking water; you need electrolytes, too. They are necessary for the proper balance of fluids inside your cells, and they play a big part in nerve and muscle function, pH balance, and blood pressure regulation. Electrolytes are minerals including sodium, potassium, calcium, magnesium, chloride, and phosphate that help carry electrical signals from your brain to the body and back through synapsis.

Signs of Dehydration:

- Dark Yellow Urine
- Dizziness
- Increased Thirst
- Muscle Cramps
- Reduced Skin Elasticity
- Tiredness

Pay attention to these signs, if you notice them, make sure to properly hydrate by drinking water with those precious electrolytes. Always keep some water with you; it's the second most critical element for survival after oxygen.

Hydration Test:

Use this method any time you or anyone else is suspected to be dehydrated.

1. Pinch the skin on the back of your hand and see how long it takes to bounce back.
2. It should bounce back immediately or within a second or two.
3. If it takes longer, you may be dehydrated.

You can buy electrolyte drink mixes, premade drinks, or make your own at home. If you buy them, check the ingredients as they may contain sugar or artificial sweeteners.

How to Properly Hydrate:

1. Buy some electrolyte drink mix or try making your own.

2. Use as directed from the manufacturer.

3. If you eat a lot of salty or processed food, you may not need any.

4. Make sure to drink around eight cups of water a day or more if it's hot and or you're sweating a lot.

LMNT

LMNT is a zero-sugar electrolyte drink mix that was started by a few health-conscious people who were eating a whole foods diet that was low in sodium and they couldn't find a good commercial electrolyte drink mix, so they decided to make their own. Their electrolyte drink mix comes in convenient single serving packets, and they offer several tasty flavors. Some of my favorites are citrus and watermelon!

LMNT's electrolyte drink mix recipe:

Ingredients:

- 16 oz–32 oz water
- 1/2 teaspoon salt (sodium & chloride)
- ¼ teaspoon cream of tartar (potassium)
- ¼ teaspoon of magnesium malate (magnesium)
- Optional
  - 2 tablespoons lime juice or ¼ cup whole raspberries
  - Dash of stevia to taste

Directions:

1. Stir or shake to mix well and serve over ice.

Chapter Summary:

If you eat a whole food diet, make sure to add plenty of salt to your food. Many people who eat healthily also try to avoid sodium, but you may not be getting enough, especially if you do a hard workout, sauna session, hot yoga, or any activity where you sweat a lot. Make sure to replenish those electrolytes if you want to stay hydrated consistently and keep your digestive system functioning optimally.

CHAPTER 11:
IMPLEMENTATION:
How to Incorporate the
Seven Key Strategies Into
Everyday Life

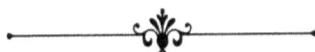

———————— ⚜ ————————

You may not need to implement all seven of the strategies discussed in this book to feel better, however, if you do take the time and incorporate them, you will be happier, healthier, and more likely to avoid future flare ups. Your gut and the rest of your body will be stronger and better able to handle small amounts of the foods that might have previously triggered an IBS attack.

In chapter 1, I told you that if you took the information in this book to heart and implemented all seven strategies, that you would be able to take back control of your life and overcome the debilitating effects of irritable bowel syndrome. You have the power to take back control of your life so you can focus on what's important to you. I can give you the information, but only you can take the steps necessary to feel better.

The Seven Key Strategies to Conquer IBS,
A Review:

One: Empower Through Education:

Understanding IBS triggers and physiological responses is crucial. Equip yourself with knowledge about what your triggers are and if you need help, consult reputable sources like our Facebook group.

Two: Personalized Diet Elimination:

Identify and avoid foods that exacerbate your symptoms. Keeping a food diary can help pinpoint specific triggers.

Three: Proactive Nourishment:

Embrace foods that promote gut health and nourish your body. Incorporate a balanced diet rich in fiber, probiotics, proteins, fats, vitamins, and minerals to strengthen your body, mind and, especially your digestive health.

Four: Home-Cooked Meals:

Preparing meals at home allows total control over ingredients and cooking methods, reducing the risk of consuming hidden IBS triggers found in processed and restaurant foods.

Five: Positive Mindset:

Mental health plays a significant role in IBS. Practices like mindfulness, stress management, and cognitive-behavioral therapy can alleviate symptoms by reducing stress-related gastrointestinal reactions.

Six: Regular Physical Activity:

Gentle, regular exercise like walking, yoga, or swimming can improve bowel function and reduce the stress that often exacerbates IBS symptoms. Resistance training will help with stress as well and is great for overall health.

Seven: Adequate Hydration:

Maintain intestinal health by drinking plenty of water. This helps digestion and can prevent the constipation often associated with IBS. If you have diarrhea, you'll need to replace fluids as well.

I was able to implement all of these strategies into my lifestyle over a few years. First, I started exercising a few days a week and meditating every morning and this gave me the confidence to start to feel good about myself. Then, I started eating more whole foods and less processed junk food products. I started tracking what I ate, and after tons of procrastination, I finally decided to try an elimination diet, I chose the carnivore diet for its simplicity. The elimination diet helped settle my IBS symptoms and once I started reincorporating other foods back into my diet, I was able to figure out what foods made my stomach hurt and gave me diarrhea, but the most valuable thing I got was something I never expected. Not eating junk food for thirty days allowed me to crush my cravings for them and I actually started craving whole foods. It was a game changer for me!

I was learning a lot about health and realized I should be hydrating, especially after a hard workout or a session in the sauna, so I started including electrolyte powders into my drinks when I needed it. I also learned from my studies that most food served at restaurants are not prepared with clean cooking methods or the ingredients I wanted to put into my body. I started cooking more at home and developing my own recipes with the right ratio of macronutrients for my needs.

One day I was reflecting on my health and realized that I had a mild case of IBS and it had vanished with my lifestyle changes. Now, when I go off script and eat foods, I know I shouldn't, I pay the price but for the most part I feel good and have regular healthy stools.

Now on the other hand Bill, the firefighter, started hydrating more, was able to reduce stress in his high stress job, and he already was very active as a fireman. The issue for him was that he was unsuccessful at changing his diet. It was hard for him to cook the right foods at the station and when they got called out on a fire, he would have to drop everything and get to work and he would end up eating fast food.

Diet is the biggest factor for getting relief from IBS, even though Bill was able to make so much progress he was ultimately unable to change his diet and he continues to suffer from IBS-C.

On the other hand, John and Barbara were able to implement all seven of the strategies and are no longer at the mercy of the toilet gods. Luckily, John narrowly avoided surgery and Barbara was able to stop the medications her doctor told her she would have to be on for the rest of her life. The hardest part for her was to stop eating junk food but the elimination diet did the trick for her.

My Recommendation To Get Better And Stay Better:

1. Start with a sixteen to twenty-four hour fast.

2. Followed by three days of only consuming homemade bone broth.

3. Then a thirty-day elimination diet of your choice

   a) Cook as much of your food yourself as you can.

4. After thirty days start eating the whole foods that you were avoiding during your elimination diet but only one at a time.

5. Keep a photo food log of everything you eat so you can correlate the food that makes you feel gross.

   a) Once identified, avoid those foods for at least three months before you try them again.

6. Continue to avoid the items on the foods to avoid list and testing to see how other foods affect you.

7. If these suggestions are too hard for you, start with working on your mental health.

Chapter Summary:

It's going to be challenging at first, but everything is when you first start something new. This method is the one thing that can stop the storm in its tracks, begin to calm your gut, and give you a life of happiness and strength.

Once you get your eating figured out, start going for walks after every meal. Even if it's only for a few minutes. It will help with your digestion and a whole lot more.

If you haven't started reducing your stress with meditation, now is the time. It may be beneficial to start speaking with a qualified mental health professional like a therapist also to help you gain a positive mindset and deal with any issues you may be holding on to.

You have the power to take back control of your life just like Barbara, John, and I did!

It may be hard, but it will be worth it, I know you can do it if you follow the advice in this book.

Take the time to cook everything you eat, avoid the foods in Chapter 5, and eat the foods listed in Chapter 6, stay hydrated, and chill out.

You got this!

CHAPTER 12:
CONQUERING IBS

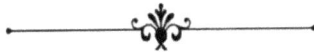

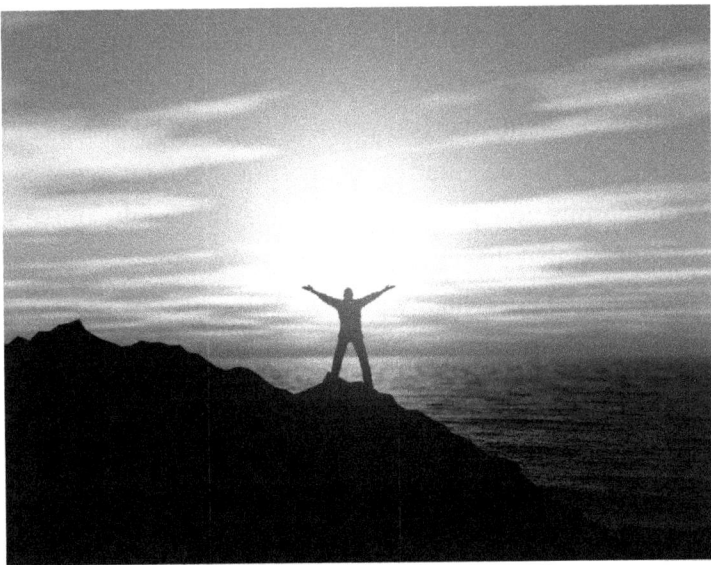

When you first started reading this book it was because you wanted to find a solution to your chronic digestive problems. By taking action and not relying on others to fix your situation, you gain the power and ability to get better and avoid the excessive trips to the bathroom and the shame associated with IBS.

You know what you need to do to feel better, all you

must do is act on the knowledge you now possess.

You can conquer IBS if you focus on healing and take it one day at a time. Start slowly by making changes to your diet and if you just can't, you will need to start working on your mental health. Speaking with a qualified mental health professional can be tremendously helpful in building up your self-confidence and self-worth to get you to a place where you can start to make the necessary changes you need to feel better and incorporate the strategies into your lifestyle.

You must start thinking of yourself as a healthy, happy person, who is free of any bowel disorders. Once you start to identify as a healthy person you will start to take on this new identity. With each and every action you take towards becoming this new person you will reaffirm to the universe and yourself that this is who you are and eventually you will become the healthy, happy person, who is free of IBS.

When, not if, you get off track, re-center yourself, take a deep breath and know there are others out there who are here to support you. They have been where you are now and have found relief from IBS. This may not be easy at first but nothing worth doing is easy at first. Remember, it will get easier, and you will start to feel better if you stick with it.

Knowledge is power and now it's up to you to utilize the knowledge you have gained from this book to find relief from IBS. Make small changes, one at a time and don't be too hard on yourself, remember you are not alone, you can do this!

"Stop your suffering and launch your healing evolution today!"

If you need additional support from people who have dealt with IBS or have questions you can join our Relief from Irritable Bowel Syndrome support group on Facebook.

www.facebook.com/groups/relieffromibs

Note From The Author:

Thank you for trusting me to help you find relief from IBS. I truly hope this book has helped you, even if you only put into use a few of the strategies, I know it will improve your life.

Now that you've made it to the end of the book, I'd love to know what you think of it. You can do this by leaving a review on Amazon. The reviews help others find the book and get relief from their IBS too.

Thank you again for your support and trust!

Joshua D. Noland

Also By Joshua D. Noland:

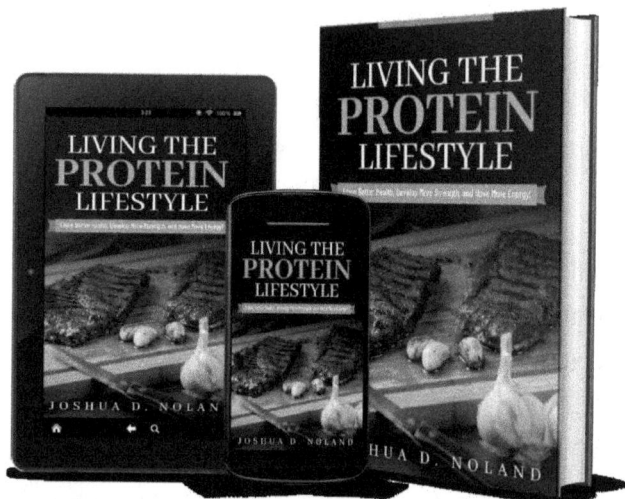

Learn how eating more protein and whole foods, staying active, and making small changes over time will create the healthy habits that will help you look and feel your best. This book will teach you how to do just that. The author lost over seventy pounds and was able to keep it off for over five years despite having knee surgery. He shares his story and the strategies and methods he uses to find lasting success, so you can too! The best part is you don't have to give up the foods you love because it's not a diet, it's a lifestyle! Whatever your preferences are, this book will teach you how to improve your health drastically.

ProteinLifestyleBook.com

Are You in Need of a Step-by-Step Approach to Improve Your Health?

My Course Offers One-on-One Coaching and a Customized Plan to Improve Your Health, One Step at a Time.

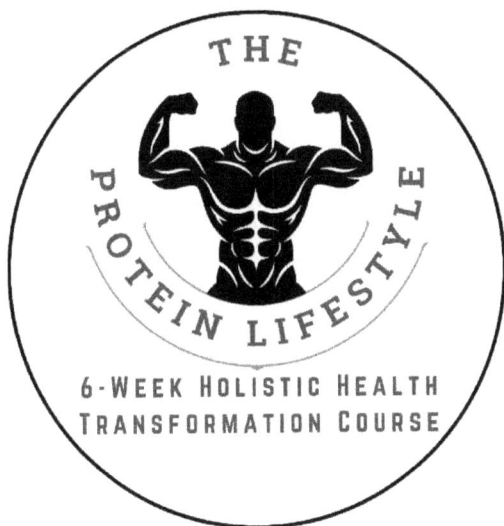

If this is all too much and you need help figuring out how to get started, the six-week holistic health transformation course is just what you need. The coaching calls and included workbook will guide you step-by-step on how to incorporate healthy habits into your life to help you feel better and find lasting success.

LaunchYourEvolution.com

BIBLIOGRAPHY

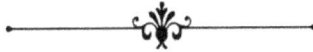

- **"Stress and the gut: pathophysiology, clinical consequences, diagnostic approach and treatment options"** by PC Konturek, T Brzozowski, and SJ Konturek (2011). This paper discusses how stress affects gut physiology, including influences on the gut mucosal barrier and interactions with the brain-gut axis, particularly in IBS.

  o https://www.jpp.krakow.pl/journal/archive/12_1 1/pdf/591_12_11_article.pdf

- **"Impact of psychological stress on irritable bowel syndrome"** by HY Qin, CW Cheng, XD Tang, and others (2014). This study explores the relationship between psychological stress and IBS, emphasizing the brain-gut axis and how various social and emotional triggers can exacerbate IBS symptoms.

  o https://www.ncbi.nlm.nih.gov/pmc/articles/PM C4202343/

- **"The place of stress and emotions in the irritable bowel syndrome"** by S Pellissier and B Bonaz (2017). This article reviews how stress and emotional factors are integrated into the management and understanding of IBS, suggesting a multifaceted approach to treatment.

- o   https://www.sciencedirect.com/science/article/pii/S0083672916300474

- **"Effect of acute physical and psychological stress on gut autonomic innervation in irritable bowel syndrome"** by CDR Murray, J Flynn, L Ratcliffe, MR Jacyna, and others (2004). The study investigates the immediate effects of stress on the gut's autonomic responses in IBS patients compared to controls.

- o   https://www.gastrojournal.org/article/S0016-5085(04)01559-8/fulltext

- **"V. Stress and irritable bowel syndrome"** by EA Mayer, BD Naliboff, L Chang, and others (2001). This paper focuses on how stress can predispose individuals to IBS, looking at the impact of chronic and acute stressors.

- o   https://journals.physiology.org/doi/full/10.1152/ajpgi.2001.280.4.G519

- Harvard Health Publishing. (2019). The ins and outs of fiber and IBS.

- Shepherd, S. J., & Gibson, P. R. (2013). The Complete Low-FODMAP Diet: A Revolutionary Plan for Managing IBS and Other Digestive Disorders.

- Monash University. (n.d.). Monash FODMAP Diet.

- Harvard T.H. Chan School of Public Health. (n.d.). Irritable Bowel Syndrome.

- Shepherd, S. J., & Gibson, P. R. (2006). Fructose malabsorption and symptoms of irritable bowel syndrome: guidelines for effective dietary management. *Journal of the American Dietetic Association*, 106(10), 1631-1639.

- Kris Gunnars. "Are Vegetable and Seed Oils Bad for Your Health?" *Healthline*. Updated June 9, 2023.

- U.S. Food and Drug Administration. Pesticide Residue Monitoring Program Fiscal Year 2016 Pesticide Report. 2018.

- Environmental Working Group: Roundup for Breakfast, Part 2, "In New Tests, Weed Killer Found in All Kids' Cereal Sampled." 2018.

- Krüger M, Schledorn P, Schrödl W, Hoppe H-W, Lutz W, Shehata AA. "Detection of Glyphosate residues in animals and humans." J Environ Anal Toxicol. 2014.

- https://www.niddk.nih.gov/health-information/health-statistics/digestive-diseases

- https://www.businessinsider.com/10-companies-control-the-food-industry-2016-9?op=1

- https://my.clevelandclinic.org/health/diseases/4342-irritable-bowel-syndrome-ibs

- https://thenaturopathicherbalist.com/herbal-actions/b-d/demulcent-2/

- https://health.clevelandclinic.org/take-control-of-ibs-with-low-fodmap-diet

- https://www.hudsonrivergi.com/blog/what-to-eat-during-an-ibs-diarrhea-flare-up

- https://aboutibs.org/what-is-ibs/

- https://health.clevelandclinic.org/low-fodmap-diet

- https://cdn.nutrition.org/article/S2475-2991(23)00512-7/fulltext

- https://www.healthline.com/nutrition/different-types-of-fiber#TOC_TITLE_HDR_3

- https://health.clevelandclinic.org/take-control-of-ibs-with-low-fodmap-diet

- www.alittlebityummy.com/blog/what-cheeses-are-low-fodmap-low-lactose/

- https://everydaynutrition.com.au/2020/01/02/is-intermittent-fasting-good-for-ibs/

www.ingramcontent.com/pod-product-compliance
Lightning Source LLC
Chambersburg PA
CBHW071426210326
41597CB00020B/3665